Fatty Liver Diet for Women

A 21-Day Liver-Friendly Meal Plan with Low-Sugar Mediterranean Recipes, Grocery Lists, and Simple Tracking

Disclaimer

This guide is provided for informational and educational purposes only and should not be interpreted as medical, nutritional, or professional advice. The author is not a licensed physician, nurse, dietitian, or mental health provider. Reading this guide does not establish a patient–provider relationship of any kind.

Always seek the guidance of a qualified healthcare professional before starting, changing, or discontinuing any supplement, diet, or lifestyle program. If you are pregnant, breastfeeding, managing a chronic medical condition, or taking prescription medications, consult your physician or pharmacist before considering any product mentioned in this guide.

The author and publisher make no representations or warranties regarding accuracy, applicability, fitness, or completeness of the information contained herein. While every effort has been made to ensure scientific accuracy and currency, medical knowledge and research evolve continually. Readers are responsible for verifying information and making decisions in consultation with licensed professionals.

Use of this guide and any information contained within it is at your own risk. The author and publisher disclaim all liability for any loss, injury, or adverse outcome that may result from the use or misuse of this material.

No supplement, diet, or practice discussed in this text is intended to diagnose, treat, cure, or prevent any disease. No outcomes or benefits are guaranteed.

Product names, supplement formulations, diet frameworks, and trademarks mentioned are the property of their respective owners and are used for identification only. Any images or illustrations that appear in related materials are licensed stock or educational placeholders.

Table of Contents

Introduction

Fatty liver disease is becoming increasingly common among adults, and women face a distinct set of metabolic and hormonal challenges that can make effective, sustainable nutrition strategies feel out of reach. Navigating dietary recommendations, deciphering conflicting information, and staying consistent can seem daunting especially when general advice fails to consider women's unique risk factors and daily routines.

Yet, for women specifically, understanding and proactively addressing fatty liver is vital: if left unchecked, fatty liver can progress, increasing the risk of serious conditions such as advanced liver disease, cardiovascular disease, and persistent fatigue that undermines quality of life.

A key factor in managing and potentially reversing fatty liver is making targeted changes to your daily eating habits. Unlike short-term or restrictive fad diets, the approach in this guide draws on the best evidence for liver health, adapting low-sugar Mediterranean principles into a 21-day plan designed both for practicality and long-term results.

While medication and medical interventions may play a role in some circumstances, this guide focuses exclusively on what you can control at home: meal composition, food selection, and daily routines. If you are managing advanced cirrhosis or require medical supervision for liver disease, consult your healthcare provider; this program does not cover prescription treatments or interventions outside of dietary guidance.

Over the next 21 days, you'll discover how meal planning and mindful eating can transform the way you approach liver health. The Mediterranean diet offers an evidence-based blueprint for supporting the liver, particularly when adapted to minimize added sugars and emphasize the right balance of whole grains, lean proteins, vegetables, healthy fats, and antioxidant-rich foods. This program is structured to give you:

- Step-by-step Mediterranean meal plans tailored for liver support and lower sugar intake
- Grocery lists and shopping strategies to simplify planning and reduce decision fatigue
- Daily and weekly meal tracking tools for greater accountability, visibility, and success
- Practical, flexible recipes that support consistency and reduce stress around food
- Self-assessment and progress check-ins to empower you throughout your journey

Throughout the guide, you will build the skills to organize your kitchen, choose the best liver-friendly ingredients, and batch-prep meals to cut down on daily cooking time. Simple checklists and food maps help you shop smarter and avoid common dietary pitfalls that can worsen liver health. Tracking systems invite you to notice subtle improvements in your energy and symptoms while pointing out when your plan may need adjustments.

Because this resource is uniquely designed for women, it spotlights considerations that matter to you: from the influence of hormonal shifts on liver metabolism to the particular patterns of symptom progression and risk factors women are more likely to face. The guide does not offer generic, one-size-fits-all advice instead, it provides a focused, actionable system designed for real results.

By the end of the 21-day program, you will not only have a strong foundation for protecting your liver but also practical routines and flexible systems to help sustain improvements well beyond this initial period. Whether you are new to Mediterranean meal planning or eager to refine your habits with proven, liver-friendly strategies, this guide equips you with the tools, know-how, and support you need to succeed starting today.

Fatty Liver in Women—Causes, Risks, and Diagnostic Criteria (Role: Fundamentals)

Understanding fatty liver disease in women begins with recognizing the distinct ways in which gender-specific biology, lifestyle factors, and the progression of nonalcoholic fatty liver disease (NAFLD) intersect. As you embark on the 21-day liver-friendly Mediterranean meal plan, grounding yourself in these fundamentals will empower informed decisions and successful, lasting change.

Gender-Specific Factors Influencing Nonalcoholic Fatty Liver Disease Incidence

NAFLD is among the fastest-rising chronic health conditions impacting women globally. Although the basic mechanism of fat accumulation in the liver unrelated to excessive alcohol use is similar for both sexes, several unique factors directly raise the risk and rate of progression for women. Chief among these are hormonal influences, metabolic differences, and specific life stages that shift liver vulnerability.

Estrogen, the primary female sex hormone, provides a protective effect on liver metabolism prior to menopause. It helps regulate how fat is stored and broken down, generally resulting in a lower risk of fatty liver disease for premenopausal women when compared to men of similar age. However, this dynamic shifts dramatically after menopause.

As estrogen levels drop, women experience an increase in metabolic risk factors such as abdominal fat accumulation, insulin resistance, and cholesterol changes all of which can accelerate the development or worsening of fatty liver disease.

Beyond ***menopause***, other stages of life like ***pregnancy*** and ***polycystic ovary syndrome (PCOS)*** can further alter liver risk profiles. PCOS is often underdiagnosed but is closely associated with increased insulin resistance, and both metabolic and reproductive hormone imbalance can foster an environment prone to fat deposition in the liver. Additionally, metabolic syndrome, a cluster of related risk factors that includes high blood pressure, abnormal cholesterol, and increased waist circumference, is particularly significant for women in their 40s and beyond.

Women's bodies metabolize nutrients, especially sugars and fats, differently than men's. As a result, certain popular diets may be less effective or even counterproductive for women seeking to reduce liver fat. A diet tailored to these underlying differences such as the structured low-sugar Mediterranean plan in this guide is specifically designed to support female metabolism and optimize liver health outcomes.

Common Symptoms, and Asymptomatic Progression Patterns in Women

Fatty liver disease is often a "silent" condition, especially in its early stages. Many women may not experience any clear, obvious symptoms until their liver has sustained significant fat buildup or inflammation. This subtlety makes it easy to miss the warning signs, delaying intervention and increasing the risk for more severe complications.

When symptoms do appear, they are frequently non-specific and may include:

- Persistent fatigue or feeling unusually tired, even with adequate rest
- Mild discomfort or dull pain in the upper right side of the abdomen
- General malaise or loss of energy
- Occasional digestive changes or bloating

However, these symptoms are not unique to fatty liver disease and can be wrongly attributed to other causes or simply to a busy lifestyle. For many women, the condition is only discovered incidentally through routine blood work or imaging studies done for unrelated health concerns.

Another pattern observed in women is a longer interval between the onset of fat accumulation and the development of more severe liver damage, such as fibrosis or cirrhosis. However, this gradual progression doesn't mean the risk is minor. Silent advancement is particularly dangerous, as the liver can sustain significant injury without obvious symptoms.

This reality highlights the value of proactive self-monitoring and regular medical check-ups for women at risk. Tracking subtle changes in energy, appetite, or even mild abdominal symptoms during this 21-day plan will be a valuable tool for catching issues before they escalate.

Diagnostic Criteria and Thresholds for Identifying Fatty Liver in Clinical Practice

A precise diagnosis of fatty liver disease in women involves both exclusion of other liver conditions (such as viral hepatitis or significant alcohol use) and confirmation of fat accumulation in the liver. There are several medical standards and thresholds clinicians use to identify, stage, and monitor NAFLD.

Diagnostically, the most widely accepted clinical threshold is the presence of greater than 5% liver fat content, as observed through imaging studies or tissue sampling. The most common tests for initial detection and assessment include:

- ***Blood tests***: Elevated levels of liver enzymes, specifically alanine aminotransferase (ALT) and aspartate aminotransferase (AST), can signal possible liver injury, though many women with NAFLD have normal enzyme values, especially in early stages.
- ***Imaging studies***: Ultrasound, transient elastography (also known as FibroScan), or MRI scans can reveal increased liver fat and, in some cases, the amount of liver stiffness, which shows if scarring (fibrosis) is present.
- ***Liver biopsy***: In rare or complex cases, a small tissue sample may be taken for microscopic analysis to confirm diagnosis and assess the degree of liver damage.

It is important to emphasize that abnormal blood results alone are not definitive for fatty liver diagnosis, especially in women, due to the common absence of symptoms and enzyme irregularities in early disease. Hence, a combination of clinical history, risk evaluation, and imaging is the gold standard in practice.

If you are using this guide and have or suspect NAFLD, regular communication with your healthcare provider particularly regarding test results during and after dietary changes—is crucial for appropriate monitoring and timely intervention.

Risk Factor Checklist Adapted for Women: Genetics, Lifestyle, Comorbidities

The foundation of successful prevention and self-management lies in knowing your personal risk profile. Women experience several distinct or magnified risk factors compared to men, some of which are modifiable through lifestyle changes and others that require heightened vigilance.

Genetics

- A family history of fatty liver disease, metabolic syndrome, type 2 diabetes, or obesity increases lifetime risk.
- Certain ethnic backgrounds ***(South Asian, Hispanic, Middle Eastern, Indigenous, Pacific Islander)*** are at higher risk due to genetic susceptibility.

Hormonal Shifts

- ***Perimenopause*** and ***menopause*** result in declining estrogen, raising the risk for fat accumulation in the liver and associated metabolic changes.
- ***PCOS*** adds risk due to chronic hormone imbalance and insulin resistance.

Lifestyle

- ***Diets*** high in processed foods, added sugars, and unhealthy fats strongly contribute to liver fat buildup.

- ***Low physical activity levels***, especially in midlife or after menopause, aggravate risk.
- ***Weight gain*** in adulthood, particularly excess central (abdominal) fat.

Comorbidities

- ***Type 2 diabetes and/or insulin resistance*** are potent risk amplifiers for NAFLD development and progression.
- ***High blood pressure, high cholesterol, and metabolic syndrome*** are often interconnected with liver risk.
- ***Sleep disturbances***, including obstructive sleep apnea, can worsen liver inflammation.

Practical steps include reviewing your family history, tracking your weight and waist circumference over time, and noting any metabolic diagnoses from your healthcare team. If you check two or more boxes on the above risk list, it is particularly important to follow the self-monitoring and dietary guidelines in this plan.

Fatty Liver Health Assessment Framework for Initial Self-Evaluation

Before diving into the 21-day meal plan, a structured self-assessment lays critical groundwork for tracking improvement. This framework emphasizes the key domains of risk awareness, symptom monitoring, and lifestyle patterns.

Step 1: Personal Risk Review

- List current and past medical conditions, focusing on diabetes, PCOS, high blood pressure, or cholesterol problems.
- Record family history of liver conditions or related metabolic diseases.

Step 2: Lifestyle Audit

- Estimate your weekly intake of processed foods, sugary snacks, and high-fat animal products.
- Track exercise frequency (aim for at least 150 minutes per week of moderate activity).

Step 3: Symptom Awareness

- Make note of any recent or recurring fatigue, mild abdominal discomfort, bloating, or digestive changes.
- Record any changes in energy levels, appetite, or mood that may be new or increasing.

Step 4: Waist Measurement

Use a measure to assess your waist circumference at the level of your belly button. A higher value (above 80 cm for women) indicates increased central obesity, a known liver risk factor.

Step 5: Laboratory and Imaging Results

- Gather copies of recent blood test results ALT, AST, and fasting glucose or HbA1c if available.
- Record the date and results of any ultrasound, elastography, or other liver imaging if completed.

This initial self-assessment not only activates your awareness but also serves as a baseline to return to after three weeks of dietary change. By developing clear, simple tracking habits facilitated by the daily logs and checklists in this guide you position yourself for early detection of meaningful improvements, such as reduced fatigue or better blood markers.

The Value of Early, Proactive Action

Women have many opportunities to intervene early and change their liver trajectory. Because many risk factors such as diet, movement, and body weight are under your influence, adopting evidence-based, manageable steps such as those in the 21-day Mediterranean plan can yield both short-term symptom relief and longer-term health protection.

While genetic or hormonal influences set the stage, they do not dictate your future. Most women, even those with significant family histories or chronic conditions, can achieve measurable benefit from focusing on a balanced, nutrient-rich diet (low in added sugars and unhealthy fats), routine movement, and consistent self-checks. The Mediterranean eating patterns featured in this plan, when aligned with tracking tools and personalized risk awareness, form a strong defense against the progression of fatty liver in women.

As you move forward, keep this assessment framework handy, and revisit it weekly. Regularly updating your symptom log, dietary scorecard, and risk checklist allows swift modification of your strategies, whether you notice improvement or encounter new challenges.

In the chapters ahead, you'll discover exactly how to build your meal plan, select ingredients, batch cook for efficiency, and monitor your progress with clarity. This foundation grounded in the understanding of your unique risks and the silent, often asymptomatic nature of fatty liver in women will guide and motivate you as you implement each dietary strategy. Remember: early, informed action is your most powerful tool for lasting liver and metabolic health.

Mediterranean Diet Principles Tailored for Liver Health (Role: Mechanisms)

Adopting a Mediterranean diet structure has garnered considerable attention for its ability to support liver health, particularly among women at risk for or living with fatty liver disease. The 21-day meal plan central to this guide draws fundamentally on Mediterranean nutrition principles, but adjusts them for the specific goal of liver fat reduction and metabolic resilience.

This chapter explains, step by step, how these dietary mechanisms work, which Mediterranean elements offer the most benefit, and how they must be adapted to limit sugars and processed fats. You will also find a categorized "foods taxonomy" to make selecting and tracking liver-friendly options effortless.

Core Mediterranean Diet Elements and Their Impact on Liver Fat Reduction

At its heart, the Mediterranean diet is a pattern rich in plant-based foods, healthy fats, moderate high-quality proteins, and minimal processed sugars or red meats. This traditional food structure originating primarily from countries bordering the Mediterranean Sea has been associated with reduced risk of chronic disease, improved cardiovascular function, and, crucially, the reversal or slowing of non-alcoholic fatty liver disease (NAFLD).

Key core elements of this eating pattern include:

- High intake of vegetables, fruits, and legumes
- Whole grains as staple carbohydrates
- Olive oil as the principal added fat
- Regular consumption of nuts and seeds
- Moderate, varied use of fish and poultry
- Low intake of red and processed meats
- Limited consumption of dairy and eggs
- Herbs and spices for flavor, with little reliance on salt
- Water as the beverage of choice

For women with NAFLD or at elevated risk particularly postmenopausal women who may have enhanced sensitivity to dietary fats and sugars this structure is notably protective. Diverse plant-based foods supply a matrix of nutrients and fiber, which together slow the absorption of sugars and regulate insulin response, cutting down the mechanisms that drive liver fat accumulation.

Several studies have shown that following a Mediterranean-style eating plan, even without strict calorie reduction, can significantly lower intrahepatic (within-liver) fat content. The balance of healthy fats (primarily monounsaturated from olive oil and polyunsaturated from nuts/fish), plentiful soluble fiber from vegetables and legumes, and the ***avoidance of quickly absorbed sugars operates through several reinforcing pathways:***

- Reduction of liver fat deposition by stabilizing blood sugar and reducing insulin spikes
- Improvement in lipid metabolism, helping the liver break down and export excess fat
- Diminished systemic inflammation, which dampens the cycles of injury in fatty liver
- Enhanced satiety, leading to spontaneous calorie moderation and less overeating.

It is these specific characteristics distinct from other popular diets high in processed foods or animal fats that make the Mediterranean approach particularly effective for liver health.

Low-Sugar Adaptations Within the Mediterranean Framework for Improved Glycemic Control

While the traditional Mediterranean diet is already lower in added sugars than many Western eating patterns, further modifications are recommended for optimizing liver recovery and glycemic control, especially for women. Chronically high sugar intake—particularly from added sugars, sodas, sweetened yogurts, and pastries is a strong independent driver of NAFLD progression. Women tend to be more sensitive to rapid swings in blood sugar and are often under more metabolic stress during key life stages such as menopause or in the presence of conditions like PCOS.

Within the 21-day plan, the Mediterranean approach is adapted by:

- Prioritizing whole fruit in small to moderate portions, consumed with meals for slower glucose absorption
- Excluding fruit juices and all sweetened beverages
- Choosing only whole grains (such as brown rice, barley, farro, or oats) over refined grains or white flours
- Skipping desserts that rely on added sugars; instead, using small amounts of naturally sweet ingredients like cinnamon-baked apples or roasted grapes (serving sizes under five grams of sugar)

- Incorporating legumes such as lentils and chickpeas, which are naturally low glycemic and help stabilize blood sugar when paired with meals
- Reading ingredient labels carefully to avoid hidden sugars in common condiments, sauces, or snack foods

These adaptations work to minimize post-meal glucose spikes, which has dual benefits: it disrupts the cycle by which excess sugar is converted into liver fat, and it helps decrease insulin resistance, a key pathological process in fatty liver disease. For women, maintaining steady blood sugar also reduces the likelihood of cravings and energy dips, supporting adherence to long-term dietary change.

Emphasis on Anti-Inflammatory and Antioxidant-Rich Foods Specific to Liver Support

Inflammation and oxidative stress are pivotal factors, not only in the buildup of liver fat, but also in its potential to progress to more serious liver injury. The Mediterranean diet provides a rich arsenal of anti-inflammatory and antioxidant nutrients, especially when composed with targeted foods supporting liver resilience.

Core anti-inflammatory and antioxidant-rich foods in this context include:

- ***Leafy greens (spinach, kale, Swiss chard)***: Packed with phytonutrients and chlorophyll, supporting detoxification
- ***Cruciferous vegetables (broccoli, Brussels sprouts, cauliflower)***: Contain natural liver-protective compounds like sulforaphane and indoles
- ***Tomatoes, red bell peppers, and eggplant***: Deliver both vitamin C and polyphenols
- ***Berries (in limited portions)***: A source of anthocyanins, which reduce oxidative stress
- ***Olive oil***: Provides vitamin E and a high concentration of monounsaturated fat, regulating inflammation
- ***Raw nuts (especially walnuts and almonds)***: Contain omega-3s and polyphenols, both protective for liver cells
- ***Garlic and onions***: Supply organosulfur compounds supporting detoxification enzymes
- ***Fresh herbs (parsley, cilantro, basil)***: High in antioxidants and replace the need for salt

Including a variety of these foods in each week of the meal plan ensures a spectrum of anti-inflammatory nutrients. For women, who may also experience increased inflammation during menopause or with underlying insulin resistance, this emphasis can translate to better liver enzyme profiles and a lower risk of progression to fibrosis

Saturated Fat and Processed Food Avoidance Criteria

A core principle for managing and reversing fatty liver is the reduction of saturated fats and processed food intake. The Mediterranean plan, when properly implemented, is designed around this avoidance strategy.

Criteria for saturated fat and processed food avoidance include:

1. Excluding or severely limiting fatty cuts of red meat (beef, pork, lamb)
2. Skipping highly processed meats (sausages, bacon, deli meats)
3. Using minimal full-fat dairy products, favoring small serves of low-fat yogurt or cheeses if included
4. Choosing plant-based oils (olive, canola, or avocado oil) over butter, ghee, coconut oil, or cream
5. Avoiding deep-fried foods, commercial baked goods, pastries, and snack chips
6. Rejecting shelf-stable items with a high list of artificial ingredients, emulsifiers, or hydrogenated oils
7. Preparing most meals from scratch to limit exposure to prepackaged sauces, convenience dinners, and ultra-processed snacks

Processed and saturated fats not only fuel liver fat buildup but also aggravate systemic inflammation and worsen insulin resistance. Women, due to their heightened metabolic sensitivity during hormonal transitions, benefit significantly from this exclusion approach, observing improved metabolic markers and leaner liver imaging results over time.

Mediterranean for Liver Support Foods Taxonomy by Food Group

To simplify meal planning and shopping, the Mediterranean diet for liver health can be broken down into clear food groups, each with uniquely supportive properties. Use the following taxonomy as a blueprint for daily and weekly meal construction and recipe variation.

1. **Vegetables:**
   - ***Focus***: At least two-thirds of plate volume at lunch and dinner
   - ***Core examples***: Leafy greens, broccoli, cauliflower, peppers, eggplant, tomatoes, carrots, onions, mushrooms, zucchini
   - ***Preparation***: Raw in salads, steamed, roasted, or sautéed in olive oil

2. **Fruits:**
   - ***Focus***: One to two small serves per day, always whole (never juice)
   - ***Core examples***: Berries, apples, pears, oranges, pomegranate, citrus, melon (in limited amounts)

- *Emphasis*: Include with meals or as a snack paired with nuts/seeds

3. **Legumes:**
   - *Focus*: Minimum of three to four servings per week
   - *Core examples*: Lentils, chickpeas, beans, split peas
   - *Emphasis*: Soups, salads, or as mains with vegetables and herbs

4. **Whole Grains:**
   - *Focus*: Replace refined carbohydrates completely
   - *Core examples*: Brown rice, whole barley, bulgur, farro, quinoa, steel-cut oats
   - *Preparation*: Cooked simply and combined with vegetables and legumes

5. **Fish and Lean Proteins:**
   - *Focus*: Oily fish two times per week, poultry or eggs in moderation
   - *Core examples*: Sardines, salmon, trout, cod, skinless chicken, turkey, eggs (1–3/week)
   - *Note*: Prioritize fish high in omega-3; avoid breaded/fried versions

6. **Tree Nuts and Seeds:**
    - ***Focus***: Small portions (a handful) four to six times weekly
    - ***Core examples***: Walnuts, almonds, pistachios, pumpkin seeds, sunflower seeds
    - ***Uses***: Added to salads, yogurt, or eaten as snacks

7. **Olive Oil and Other Plant Oils:**
    - ***Focus***: Main source of added fat
    - ***Criteria***: Use extra-virgin when possible; limit total added oils to 1–3 tablespoons per day

8. **Dairy (if included):**
    - ***Focus***: Low-fat and minimally processed
    - ***Core examples***: Plain Greek yogurt, kefir
    - ***Note***: Avoid sweetened or flavored varieties

9. **Herbs, Spices, and Flavorings:**
    - ***Focus***: Substitute for salt and sauces
    - ***Use***: Fresh or dried basil, oregano, mint, coriander, cumin, turmeric, cinnamon

10. **Beverages:**
    - ***Focus***: Water (main), herbal teas
    - ***Avoid***: Sugar-sweetened sodas, processed fruit juices, even low-calorie/diet drinks

This taxonomy allows women to rotate foods to suit personal preference and seasonal availability, while always staying within the boundaries shown to support liver function and metabolic health.

The strength of the Mediterranean approach lies in its synergistic design: every food group, when chosen and prepared correctly, acts in concert to lower liver fat, reduce inflammation, control blood sugar, and improve overall vitality. Compared to restrictive fad diets or highly processed modern eating patterns, the Mediterranean framework offers not just a scientifically grounded foundation, but also diversity, enjoyment, and adaptability.

Using the principles in this chapter, you are equipped to implement the 21-day plan in a manner finely tuned to women's metabolic realities and liver health priorities. As you proceed to meal planning and practical recipe selection, return to these core mechanisms as the rationale for every recommended ingredient, swap, and menu choice. Small incremental changes tracking vegetables, sugar intake, and avoidance of processed foods yield compounding benefits for your liver, energy, and long-term health trajectory.

Embracing this holistic, Mediterranean-inspired pattern, and tailoring it for low-sugar, anti-inflammatory, and antioxidant emphasis, paves the way for sustainable change delivering both near-term improvements and the best possible defense against fatty liver disease progression.

Building Your 21-Day Liver-Friendly Meal Structure (Role: Systems)

The foundation of a successful liver-friendly Mediterranean meal plan lies in creating balanced meals that consistently maintain low sugar intake throughout the day. For women with or at risk of fatty liver disease, this is crucial, as female bodies often react more rapidly to sugar fluctuations, especially during metabolic stress or hormonal changes. Each meal breakfast, lunch, and dinner should be constructed to stabilize blood sugar, reduce added and hidden sugars, and support liver healing.

A practical meal structure includes the following principles:

Breakfast should be rich in fiber, healthy fats, and moderate protein, but low in sugars: Skip sweetened cereals, pastries, and juices in favor of steel-cut oats with nuts, Greek yogurt topped with a few berries, or an omelet with greens and a drizzle of olive oil.

Lunch and dinner focus on plates dominated by non-starchy vegetables (at least half the meal's volume), moderate portions of lean protein (such as fish, legumes, or skinless poultry), and small servings of whole grains (like brown rice or barley). Emphasize olive oil as the primary fat and use fresh herbs and spices for flavor.

Snacks are optional but, if needed, should also align with these guidelines: raw nuts, sliced vegetables with hummus, or a small apple paired with pumpkin seeds.

To consistently maintain a low sugar profile, plan meals using only whole fruits in modest amounts, completely avoid fruit juices or sweetened beverages, and be vigilant about hidden sugars in condiments or packaged products. When in doubt, assemble your meal with an abundance of plant-based ingredients, as fiber-rich foods slow sugar absorption and protect against rapid spikes.

Weekly meal rotation system for nutrient variety and liver protection

Monotony is the enemy of both nutritional balance and sustainable habit formation. Repeating the same foods day after day can lead to nutrient gaps, taste fatigue, and ultimately, lower adherence to a liver-friendly plan. Instead, use a weekly meal rotation system cycling through diverse vegetables, proteins, whole grains, and flavorings to ensure comprehensive nutrient coverage and ongoing support for liver protection.

Variety within the Mediterranean pattern also delivers a wider array of antioxidants, phytonutrients, and fibers, all of which contribute directly to liver healing. For example, rotating between different leafy greens (kale, spinach, Swiss chard), whole grains (quinoa, barley, farro), legumes (lentils, chickpeas, beans), and fish or plant-based proteins across the week boosts the protective and detoxifying effects of your meal structure.

Each week, choose at least one "new" ingredient in each category:

- ***Vegetables***: Swap broccoli for Brussels sprouts, or bell peppers for zucchini
- ***Proteins***: Alternate chickpeas with lentils or flank a meal with salmon rather than chicken
- ***Grains***: Rotate brown rice with quinoa or bulgur
- ***Herbs and spices***: Use fresh basil one week, fresh mint or cilantro the next

Aim for the "rainbow" variety; more color means more unique nutrients. Not only does this make meals more enjoyable, but it also maximizes different micronutrients and antioxidants known to combat liver inflammation and fat accumulation. When planning your week, batch-prep certain ingredients (like a big tray of roasted mixed vegetables) but serve them with different herbs, proteins, or grains on subsequent days.

Portion size guidelines and visual aids for meal composition

Mindful portion sizing is fundamental to both liver health and steady energy levels. Too large a portion, even of wholesome foods, can disrupt the balance needed for sustainable improvement. For effective and practical application:

- ***Vegetables***: Should fill at least half your plate, focusing on non-starchy, preferably raw, steamed, or roasted with a dash of olive oil.
- ***Protein***: Target one-quarter of your plate—visualize a serving about the size and thickness of your palm, or roughly 90–120 grams cooked.
- ***Whole grains or starchy vegetables***: Limit to one-quarter of your plate, equivalent to about half a cup cooked (the size of a small cupped hand).
- ***Healthy fats***: Use sparingly (1–2 tablespoons of olive oil or a small handful of nuts/seeds).
- ***Fruit***: If eaten at a meal, confine to a small portion, complementing the meal—like a half-cup of berries or one small apple.

Visual cues make daily planning easy and help prevent over- or under-consumption, which can either slow progress or leave you unsatisfied. **A standard dinner plate measures about 23 cm (9 in) wide:**

- Draw an invisible line down the middle; one side is all colorful vegetables.
- Divide the remaining half into two—one for lean protein, the other for whole grains.
- Place some sliced fruit or a portion of nuts on the side, not piled in with other foods.

This visual template works for both home-prepared and restaurant meals, empowering quick, healthy decisions even on busy days.

Core meal-building blocks checklist for rapid daily planning

To streamline daily meal prep and ensure every plate meets low-sugar Mediterranean-liver criteria, use the following core checklist. **Build your meals by ticking off each section:**

1. At least two types of non-starchy vegetables (raw or cooked)
2. Moderate: serving of lean protein (fish, legumes, poultry, or eggs in moderation—avoid fried)
3. One portion of whole grains or fiber-rich carbohydrate (quinoa, barley, steel-cut oats, brown rice, or roasted sweet potato)

4. A small amount of healthy fat (extra-virgin olive oil, avocado, or a handful of nuts/seeds)
5. One small portion of fruit, if desired, paired with a protein or fat source to blunt sugar absorption
6. Flavor boosters fresh herbs, spices, citrus, vinegar (skip creamy or sweetened dressings)

Every main meal should check all (or most) of these boxes. If you skip grains at breakfast in favor of extra veggies, try to include whole grains at lunch. If you forgo animal protein at lunch, add chickpeas or beans. Balance and variety, anchored to this list, keep the diet nutrient-rich and interesting.

Sample Weekly Meal Pattern Table for three baseline menus

To put the system into action, the following is a sample meal pattern table for a week, rotating three foundation menus across the 21 days. Each pattern meets the Mediterranean, low-sugar, and liver-healing requirements for women. Use this as a baseline, then swap items for seasonal or preferred alternatives using earlier checklists.

Menu 1: "Greens & Grains Focus"

- ***Breakfast***: Spinach and mushroom omelet with sliced tomato; 1/4 avocado; herbal tea

- ***Lunch***: Mixed greens salad with grilled chicken, chickpeas, red bell pepper, and farro; lemon-olive oil dressing
- ***Dinner***: Roasted salmon with broccoli, cauliflower, and brown rice; sprinkle of toasted walnuts

Menu 2: "Legume & Berry Boost"

- ***Breakfast***: Plain Greek yogurt with a small portion of mixed berries and raw pumpkin seeds, cinnamon
- ***Lunch***: Lentil and vegetable stew with kale; side of whole-grain toast; apple slices
- ***Dinner***: Stir-fried mixed vegetables (eggplant, peppers, zucchini) with tofu or shrimp over quinoa; mint garnish

Menu 3: "Classic Mediterranean"

- ***Breakfast***: Oats soaked overnight with finely diced apple, cinnamon, chia seeds, and almond slivers
- ***Lunch***: Chickpea tabbouleh salad (parsley, tomato, cucumber, lemon, olive oil); roast chicken breast
- ***Dinner***: Baked cod with Mediterranean vegetable medley (tomatoes, onions, peppers, olives), served with barley

Each menu is built around core meal-building blocks, rotating proteins and grains while keeping vegetables central. Rotate these menus through the week for instance, Menu 1 on Monday and Thursday, Menu 2 on Tuesday and Friday, Menu

3 on Wednesday and Saturday, with Sunday for using up leftovers or making a favorite dish from the week's patterns.

Weekly variety is achieved not just by menu, but via ingredient swaps change salmon for trout, kale for spinach, or lentils for chickpeas as the seasons and your preferences dictate. This structure maintains balance, prevents overreliance on any one ingredient, and maximizes nutrient breadth, all while keeping sugar low and liver protection high.

Expanded practical tips for implementing your meal system

- ***Plan and batch-prep a mix of raw and roasted vegetables early in the week***. Store separately so they can be added to salads, omelets, soups, or grain bowls as needed.
- ***Pre-portion nuts and seeds for snacks to prevent unintentional overeating***: Keep servings to a small handful each.
- ***Roast a tray of root vegetables*** (carrots, squash, onions) to serve hot with dinner or cold in salads.
- ***Keep a few hard-boiled eggs***: Tins of fish in water or olive oil, and cooked lentils on hand for fast protein options.
- ***Always pair fruits with a fat or protein***: Apple with almond butter, berries in yogurt, orange slices with chopped walnuts.

- ***Use herbs liberally and experiment weekly***: Cilantro, basil, dill, and parsley can all elevate simple foods.

Troubleshooting boundary conditions

- If you are especially sensitive to sugars, omit fruit from breakfast and opt for more veggies or a little extra protein, adding fruit later in the day (with lunch or a snack).
- For extra-busy days, combine pre-cooked grains with canned legumes, chopped pre-washed greens, and a store-bought rotisserie chicken (skin removed) dress with olive oil, lemon, and herbs.
- When eating out, scan the menu for any dish where you can identify most of your building blocks in their natural state (grilled fish, side of vegetables, salad base, olive oil dressing).
- Avoid all sources of sweetened beverages or fruit juices. If craving something different to drink, try cold-brewed herbal teas, infused water (with slices of cucumber, lemon, or berries), or sparkling water with a splash of fresh citrus.

The advantage of this systematic approach is its adaptability: as you become more comfortable with these frameworks, you can tailor your 21-day plan to fit changing routines, special events, or shifting seasonal produce. Remember, the goal isn't perfection, but high adherence to principles known to support liver healing, minimize sugar exposure, and provide broad nutrition.

Consider keeping a visual checklist near your meal prep area. With repetition, these steps will become intuitive, and your confidence in building liver-friendly Mediterranean meals will increase.

Construct your meal plan in a dynamic, rotating, and balanced manner to establish a strong, adaptable foundation for ongoing liver wellness, metabolic resilience, and daily satisfaction pursue not just symptom management, but real, positive transformation in your liver health.

Low-Sugar Mediterranean Recipes for Each Meal (Role: Application)

Applying a liver-friendly, low-sugar Mediterranean meal plan hinges on transforming foundational dietary knowledge into satisfying, realistic daily choices. For women managing fatty liver, this means streamlining meal preparation and cooking to routinely focus on ingredients proven to lower sugar exposure and support liver repair.

This chapter moves beyond principles to hands-on strategies, equipping you with clear templates, practical food pairings, substitution tips, and a robust recipe index designed for both simplicity and nutrient breadth.

Breakfast formula templates with low-glycemic ingredients

A liver-supportive breakfast should deliver slow-burning energy, support stable blood sugar, and meet Mediterranean standards. The goal is to fill your morning plate with foods that are naturally low on the glycemic index, minimizing both sugars and rapid starch breakdown. For women with fatty liver, this reduces metabolic stress during a sensitive window of the day, when overnight fasting ends and hormonal balance can impact how the liver processes glucose.

The Mediterranean approach calls for a blend of protein, healthy fats, and natural fibers. Key template components include:

- ***Steel-cut or traditional rolled oats***: Provides soluble fiber and slow energy; top with a minimal amount of chopped nuts, seeds (chia, pumpkin, or sunflower), and a sprinkling of cinnamon.
- ***Greek yogurt, plain and full-fat or low-fat (unsweetened)***: Pairs well with a handful of berries or a few slices of kiwi for antioxidants and flavor.
- ***Egg-based dishes***: Omelets or frittatas cooked with olive oil, chopped spinach, onions, tomatoes, and mushrooms deliver proteins and phytonutrients.
- ***Whole grain toast or small pita***: If included, use in moderation and top with half a mashed avocado, sliced tomato, and cracked black pepper.
- ***Sautéed greens***: Quickly cook kale, chard, or spinach in olive oil and lemon juice; serve as a side or mixed into eggs.

These foundations can be rotated to avoid monotony and are easily adjusted for preference and seasonal ingredients. Always limit or skip added sweeteners, and if using fruit, favor berries, green apple slices, or a few pomegranate seeds keeping the portion under half a cup. Milk alternatives (such as unsweetened almond or oat milk) can be used in porridge or smoothies, but always verify added sugar is absent in the ingredient list.

Practical breakfast ideas within this framework include:

- ***Mushroom and arugula omelet***, sliced tomato, and a drizzle of olive oil
- ***Plain Greek yogurt*** with 1/2 cup blackberries and 1 tablespoon sunflower seeds
- ***Overnight oats*** with diced green apple, chia seeds, and cinnamon
- ***Sautéed spinach*** folded with scrambled eggs, side of cherry tomatoes

These options avoid the sugar spikes of processed cereals, pastries, and sweetened breakfast drinks, facilitating a gentle start to your metabolism and prolonged satiety.

Protein-focused lunches with fiber-rich vegetables and grain substitutes

Lunchtime is crucial for reinforcing liver-friendly eating routines. Here, balancing lean proteins, a rainbow of fiber-rich vegetables, and minimizing traditional starches (such as white bread and rice) is especially impactful for women's metabolic health and liver fat reduction.

To construct a satisfying, Mediterranean-style lunch:

- ***Start with two or more types of non-starchy vegetables***. These can be raw, roasted, or steamed—think mixed greens, peppers, carrots, cucumbers, or leftover roasted Brussels sprouts.
- ***Add a protein (80–120 grams cooked)***: grilled chicken breast, tinned tuna (in olive oil or water), salmon, hard-boiled eggs, baked tofu, or legumes (chickpeas, lentils, cannellini beans).
- ***For grains***: substitute with high-fiber, low-glycemic options—quinoa, barley, or farro are ideal, but keep portions small (1/2 cup cooked).
- ***Include healthy fats***: olives, a tablespoon of extra-virgin olive oil drizzled as dressing, or a small portion of feta or goat cheese.
- ***Add flavor***: fresh herbs, lemon, garlic, and spices (cumin, paprika, fresh basil) amplify flavor without extra calories or sugars.

Lunch bowl formula:

- *Base*: 1–2 cups mixed greens + ½ cup cooked vegetables (e.g., broccoli, roasted cauliflower, zucchini)
- *Protein*: 90g poached salmon, grilled chicken, or ½ cup cooked chickpeas
- *Grains*: ½ cup quinoa or barley or, if preferred, double the vegetables and forgo grains

- *Fat*: 6–8 olives or 1 tablespoon seeds/nuts or 1 tablespoon olive oil

Creative lunch combinations from this template:

1. Mixed salad with leafy greens, roasted bell peppers, chickpeas, lemon-tahini dressing, topped with fresh parsley
2. Grilled chicken atop cooked farro, arugula, and cherry tomatoes, olives, basil, and vinaigrette
3. Lentil salad with cucumbers, tomatoes, scallions, and mint, dressed in olive oil-lemon
4. Poached salmon with a side of roasted eggplant, zucchini, and a spoonful of hummus

Adjust lunch compositions depending on your schedule and appetite. Batch-preparing proteins and vegetables in advance can cut down on mid-week prep and help maintain adherence.

Dinner pairings prioritizing lean proteins, legumes, and healthy fats

Dinner should reinforce Mediterranean and liver-friendly patterns, with emphasis on lean protein and filling, fiber-rich sides. Compared to lunch, the evening meal is a prime opportunity to increase vegetable intake, swap out heavier starches for legumes, and round out the day's healthy fat consumption.

Dinner composition best practices:

- Prioritize lean animal or plant proteins: baked or grilled fish, skinless poultry, legumes, or tofu.
- Fill half the plate with a warm or roasted vegetable medley; mix at least three colors or varieties (e.g., broccoli, red onion, carrot).
- For a hearty side, favor legumes, lentils or chickpea stews, or a warm bean salad rather than white rice or pasta.
- Use extra-virgin olive oil for roasting or drizzling; limit cheese to a light garnish.
- For flavor, leverage herbs, garlic, finely diced shallots, and citrus zest.

Sample dinner pairings:

1. Baked cod with a tray of Mediterranean vegetables (onion, eggplant, tomato, zucchini) tossed in olive oil and fresh thyme, with a side of lemony lentil salad.
2. Grilled turkey breast slices with steamed asparagus, roasted peppers, and a tomato-cucumber salad.
3. White bean stew simmered with spinach, chopped tomatoes, and garlic, finished with olive oil.
4. Saffron cauliflower "rice" (pulled in a food processor and sautéed lightly) topped with grilled shrimp and wilted kale.

Lean proteins and legumes steady evening blood sugar levels, and extra veggies help satisfy while reducing the tendency to snack on sugary foods later at night.

Snack swaps and desserts under five grams of sugar per serving

Smart snacking not only curbs hunger but also supports a steady metabolism and helps maintain low daily sugar intake. For this meal plan, snacks and desserts should never exceed five grams of sugar per serving, and ideally contribute extra fiber or phytonutrients, not just empty calories.

Snack and dessert suggestions:

- A small handful of raw or lightly roasted nuts and seeds (almonds, walnuts, pumpkin seeds), pre-portioned to prevent overconsumption.
- Hummus or white bean dip with sliced bell pepper, cucumber, or celery sticks.
- One small apple or pear, sliced and paired with a tablespoon of almond butter or a few walnuts.
- Greek yogurt (plain, unsweetened) mixed with cinnamon and a few chopped strawberries.
- Roasted chickpeas with paprika, olive oil, and a pinch of sea salt—a fiber- and protein-rich alternative to chips or crackers.

- Homemade energy bites (blended dates, oats, nuts, unsweetened cocoa)—limit to one per serving so total sugar remains low.
- Baked apple, cored and filled with cinnamon and chopped walnuts, roasted with no added sugars.

For special treats:

- Dark chocolate (70% cacao or higher), in squares of 5 grams or less per snack serving.
- Ricotta cheese mixed with lemon zest, vanilla, and a spoonful of chia seeds—chill and serve with a few berries as a spoon dessert.

These snacks and desserts deliver continuous energy without the crash of sugar-laden foods, while providing important micronutrients, minerals, and healthy fats.

15-Recipe Quick Reference Index for simple modifications and substitutions

To empower rapid adaptation within the meal plan, here's a 15-recipe reference—templates easily modifiable to suit personal tastes, seasonal produce, or dietary needs. Each recipe is designed to preserve low sugar and Mediterranean integrity for women with fatty liver.

Breakfast

Greek Yogurt Parfait

Ingredients:

- 1 cup plain Greek yogurt
- 1/2 cup mixed berries (such as blueberries, raspberries, or strawberries)
- 2 tablespoons pumpkin seeds (or substitute chia seeds or sunflower seeds)

Instructions:

1. Spoon half of the yogurt into a glass or bowl.
2. Add half of the berries and half of the seeds.
3. Layer the remaining yogurt, berries, and seeds on top.
4. Serve immediately.

Savory Steel-Cut Oat Bowl

Ingredients:

- 1/2 cup steel-cut oats
- 1 cup water
- 1/2 cup steamed spinach (or other greens)
- 1 poached egg
- 1 teaspoon olive oil
- Salt and pepper to taste

Instructions:

1. Cook steel-cut oats according to package instructions.
2. Steam spinach or greens while oats cook.
3. Combine cooked oats and steamed greens in a bowl.
4. Top with a poached egg.
5. Drizzle with olive oil and season with salt and pepper.

Mediterranean Veggie Omelet

Ingredients:

- 2 eggs
- 1/4 cup chopped tomatoes
- 2 tablespoons chopped onions
- 1 tablespoon chopped fresh basil
- 2 tablespoons feta cheese (or substitute goat cheese)
- Salt and pepper to taste

Instructions:

1. Beat eggs in a bowl and season with salt and pepper.
2. Heat a non-stick skillet over medium heat and pour in eggs.
3. Add tomatoes, onions, and basil evenly over the eggs.
4. Sprinkle with feta or goat cheese.
5. Cook until eggs are set, then fold and serve.

Avocado Toast

Ingredients:

- 1 slice whole grain bread, toasted
- 1/2 ripe avocado, mashed
- 2 thinly sliced radishes
- 1 tablespoon mixed seeds (sunflower, pumpkin, or chia)
- Optional: sautéed greens as a substitute for radish

Instructions:

1. Toast the bread to your liking.
2. Spread mashed avocado over the toast.
3. Top with radish slices and sprinkle with seeds (or sautéed greens if desired).
4. Serve immediately.

Overnight Berry Oats

Ingredients:

- 1/2 cup rolled oats
- 1 tablespoon chia seeds
- 1 cup almond milk
- 1/2 cup blackberries or sliced kiwi

Instructions:

1. In a jar or bowl, combine oats, chia seeds, and almond milk.
2. Stir well, cover, and refrigerate overnight.
3. In the morning, top with blackberries or kiwi.
4. Serve chilled.

Lunch

Rainbow Chickpea Salad

Ingredients:

- 1 can chickpeas, drained and rinsed
- 1 cup assorted chopped vegetables (such as bell peppers, cucumber, cherry tomatoes)
- 2 tbsp olive oil
- Juice of 1 lemon
- Salt and pepper to taste
- Fresh herbs (such as parsley or cilantro), optional

Instructions:

1. In a large bowl, combine chickpeas and chopped vegetables.
2. Drizzle with olive oil and lemon juice.
3. Season with salt, pepper, and fresh herbs if using.
4. Toss to combine. Swap in different beans or herbs as desired.

Roasted Vegetable Grain Bowl

Ingredients:

- 2 cups assorted seasonal vegetables (such as sweet potato, zucchini, broccoli), chopped
- 1 tbsp olive oil
- 1 cup cooked quinoa (substitute with farro or barley if preferred)
- 2 tbsp fresh herbs (such as basil or parsley)
- Salt and pepper to taste

Instructions:

1. Preheat the oven to 400°F (200°C).
2. Toss vegetables with olive oil, salt, and pepper. Spread on a baking sheet.
3. Roast for 20-25 minutes until tender and golden.
4. Combine roasted vegetables with cooked quinoa and fresh herbs.
5. Serve warm or at room temperature. Substitute grains as desired.

Tuna Salad Lettuce Wraps

Ingredients:

- 1 can tuna, drained (or tinned mackerel/salmon)
- 1 stalk celery, finely chopped
- 2 tbsp Greek yogurt
- 1 tsp mustard
- Salt and pepper to taste
- Crisp lettuce leaves (such as romaine or butter lettuce)

Instructions:

1. In a bowl, mix tuna, celery, Greek yogurt, and mustard.
2. Season with salt and pepper.
3. Spoon the mixture into lettuce leaves.
4. Serve immediately. Swap tuna for mackerel or salmon if desired.

Mediterranean Lentil Soup

Ingredients:

- 1 cup dried lentils, rinsed
- 1 carrot, diced
- 1 celery stalk, diced
- 1 can diced tomatoes
- 1 tsp mixed dried herbs (such as oregano, thyme)
- 1 tsp paprika
- 4 cups vegetable broth
- Salt and pepper to taste

Instructions:

1. In a pot, combine lentils, carrot, celery, diced tomatoes, herbs, paprika, and broth.
2. Bring to a boil, then reduce heat and simmer for 30-35 minutes until lentils are tender.
3. Season with salt and pepper.
4. Blend for a smooth texture or leave chunky for variety.

Grilled Chicken and Arugula Plate

Ingredients:

- 1 grilled chicken breast, sliced
- 2 cups arugula (or substitute with spinach)
- 1 orange, segmented (optional)
- 1/4 cup olives
- 2 tbsp toasted nuts (optional)
- 1 tbsp olive oil
- Salt and pepper to taste

Instructions:

1. Arrange arugula (or spinach) on a plate.
2. Top with sliced grilled chicken, orange segments, olives, and nuts if using.
3. Drizzle with olive oil and season with salt and pepper.
4. Serve immediately. Substitute greens or add nuts as desired.

Baked Fish with Vegetable Medley

Ingredients:

- Fish fillets (any white fish, or substitute with tofu for vegetarian)
- Tomatoes, sliced
- Olives, pitted and sliced
- Onions, thinly sliced

Instructions:

1. Preheat the oven to 375°F (190°C).
2. Place fish fillets or tofu in a baking dish.
3. Layer tomatoes, olives, and onions over the fish.
4. Season with salt, pepper, and herbs as desired.
5. Bake for 20–25 minutes, until fish is cooked through or tofu is heated.

Bean and Spinach Stew

Ingredients:

- Beans (any legume, such as cannellini, chickpeas, or lentils)
- Fresh spinach (or substitute with kale or Swiss chard)
- Garlic, minced
- Onion, chopped

Instructions:

1. In a pot, sauté onion and garlic until fragrant.
2. Add beans and greens (spinach, kale, or chard).
3. Pour in enough water or broth to cover the ingredients.
4. Simmer for 15–20 minutes, until the greens are tender.
5. Season to taste with salt, pepper, and herbs.

Herbed Turkey Skewers

Ingredients:

- Ground turkey
- Zucchini, cut into chunks
- Bell peppers, cut into chunks
- Fresh or dried herbs (such as parsley, oregano, or thyme)
- Salt and pepper

Instructions:

1. In a bowl, mix ground turkey with herbs, salt, and pepper.
2. Form turkey mixture into sausage-like shapes around skewers.
3. Alternate threading zucchini and pepper chunks onto skewers.
4. Grill or broil skewers for 10–12 minutes, turning occasionally, until turkey is cooked through.

Eggplant and Tomato Casserole

Ingredients:

- Eggplant, sliced
- Tomato sauce (no added sugars)
- Fresh herbs (such as basil or oregano)
- Cheese (optional, for topping)

Instructions:

1. Preheat the oven to 375°F (190°C).
2. Bake eggplant slices until tender.
3. In a casserole dish, layer baked eggplant and tomato sauce.
4. Sprinkle fresh herbs between layers.
5. Top with a sprinkle of cheese if desired.
6. Bake for 15–20 minutes, until bubbling and heated through.

Quinoa-Stuffed Bell Peppers

Ingredients:

- Bell peppers, halved and seeded
- Cooked quinoa
- Chickpeas
- Diced tomato
- Onion, chopped
- Fresh parsley, chopped

Instructions:

1. Preheat the oven to 375°F (190°C).
2. Mix cooked quinoa, chickpeas, diced tomato, onion, and parsley in a bowl.
3. Fill bell pepper halves with quinoa mixture.
4. Place stuffed peppers in a baking dish.
5. Bake for 25–30 minutes, until peppers are tender.

Modification strategies:

- Vegetarians can replace animal proteins with legumes, tofu, or tempeh in any lunch or dinner recipe.
- For gluten intolerance, always use gluten-free grains (quinoa, rice) and verify ingredient labels for cross-contamination.
- Ingredients like fresh herbs, nuts, and seeds can be swapped based on season and preference.
- Omit or exchange dairy components (yogurt, cheese) for unsweetened plant-based alternatives as needed.

This index serves as a map for effortless week-to-week meal variety. Pick a recipe, swap a grain or protein, change herbs or vegetables, flexibility is built in while retaining core liver-friendly elements.

Incorporating low-sugar Mediterranean recipes into your daily routine is a powerful, practical step for women seeking to reverse fatty liver and restore metabolic health. These frameworks and recipes prove that eating for liver wellness is far from restrictive; it is colorful, flavorful, varied, and sustainable for life. By referring to these adaptable meal templates daily, you maintain momentum toward lasting, positive change.

Liver-Safe Ingredient Selection and Pantry Setup (Role: Tools)

Liver health hinges as much on the everyday choices in your kitchen cabinets as it does on meal planning and preparation. For women managing fatty liver, creating a carefully stocked pantry, fridge, and freezer is more than a convenience; it is a cornerstone of success. This chapter serves as your toolkit for strategically selecting, organizing, and managing ingredients that promote liver repair, minimize sugar, and sustain Mediterranean eating with confidence and ease. You will find research-based lists, actionable inventories, label-reading skills, and seasonal shopping strategies to optimize every aspect of your food environment for liver support.

List of Liver-Supportive Foods to Always Keep on Hand

The foods you choose to stock and reach for daily are the backbone of your liver-friendly Mediterranean meal plan. Prioritizing whole, minimally processed ingredients that support liver function facilitates both meal preparation and long-term health improvements. The following categories define essential liver-supportive foods for your ongoing kitchen inventory:

1. ***Vegetables***: Aim to keep a vibrant assortment, especially leafy greens (spinach, kale, arugula, Swiss chard), cruciferous varieties (broccoli, cauliflower, Brussels sprouts), and versatile staples (peppers, zucchini, eggplant, tomatoes, onions, garlic). These vegetables are high in fiber, antioxidants, and phytonutrients known to reduce liver inflammation and assist in fat metabolism.
2. ***Fruits***: Stock fresh or frozen berries (blueberries, strawberries, raspberries), citrus (lemons, oranges), green apples, and pomegranates. These deliver antioxidants with a lower glycemic load compared to sweeter, tropical fruits. Keep portions moderate to avoid excess sugars.
3. ***Legumes***: Chickpeas, lentils, cannellini beans, black beans, and split peas add fiber, plant-based protein, and help maintain stable blood sugar—key for liver health and female hormone balance.
4. ***Whole Grains***: Choose minimally processed grains like oats, quinoa, barley, farro, or brown rice. These offer complex carbs and fiber, slowly digested to reduce glycemic impact. Strictly avoid ultra-processed grain products.
5. ***Nuts and Seeds***: Almonds, walnuts, sunflower seeds, chia, and pumpkin seeds should be stored raw or

lightly roasted without added salt or sugar. They contribute healthy fats, vitamin E, and anti-inflammatory benefits.

6. ***Healthy Fats***: Always have extra-virgin olive oil, as it is central to both Mediterranean cuisine and liver protection. Also keep modest amounts of avocado and small servings of olives for snacks or salads.
7. ***Lean Proteins***: Prioritize skinless poultry, fish (especially fatty types like salmon or sardines rich in omega-3), and eggs. Plant-based proteins especially pulses should also be rotation staples.
8. ***Herbs and Spices***: Rosemary, basil, thyme, oregano, parsley, dill, mint, garlic, and ground spices offer flavor without sodium or sugar and provide added antioxidants.
9. ***Dairy***: Plain Greek yogurt and small quantities of reduced-fat cheeses (feta, ricotta, goat cheese) add protein and calcium. Choose unsweetened, minimally processed options to avoid hidden sugars.

Keeping these foods as the backbone of your kitchen helps establish a strong foundation for any meal or snack to align with liver-protective, female-oriented Mediterranean eating.

Pantry, Fridge, and Freezer Inventory Templates for Meal Prep Efficiency

Efficient meal prep starts with knowing exactly what's on hand. These templates will streamline your cooking, cut waste, and reduce the stress of last-minute grocery runs. Use them as checklists to update weekly, making adjustments for household size or menu preferences.

Pantry Inventory

- Whole grains: Oats, quinoa, barley, brown rice, farro
- Dried/canned legumes: Chickpeas, lentils, black beans, cannellini beans
- Olive oil and vinegars (balsamic, red wine, apple cider)
- Canned tomatoes (no added sugar/salt)
- Tinned fish (tuna, salmon, sardines in water or olive oil)
- Raw, unsalted nuts and seeds
- Dried herbs and spices: Basil, oregano, garlic, paprika, rosemary, thyme
- Low-sodium vegetable or chicken broth
- Whole grain crackers (if using) verify ingredient list for added sugars

Fridge Inventory

- Fresh vegetables (rotated seasonally)
- Leafy greens (spinach, arugula, kale, Swiss chard)

- Eggs
- Unsweetened Greek yogurt
- Fresh herbs
- Lemons and oranges
- Low-fat cheeses (feta, ricotta, cottage cheese)
- Avocados

Freezer Inventory

- Mixed berries, cherries, or sliced green apples (for smoothies/oats)
- Mixed vegetables (as backup or for quick stir-fries)
- Pre-cooked beans or grains (portion in bags/containers)
- Fish filets or lean poultry (portion control)
- Homemade bean stews or soups (in single-meal batches)

Consider posting copies of these templates on your pantry or fridge doors, checking off items as you use them and forming the basis of your weekly shopping lists.

Checklist for Reading Food Labels to Spot Hidden Sugars and Unhealthy Fats

Optimizing your pantry isn't just about what to add, but also about what to avoid. For women with fatty liver, vigilance about hidden sugars, refined flours, and unhealthy fats is crucial to prevent undermining your progress. Use the following checklist every time you shop for packaged or processed foods:

1. ***Check for Added Sugars***: Scan the ingredients list, not just the nutrition panel; added sugars appear under many names (e.g., sucrose, fructose, honey, maple syrup, cane juice). The lower on the list, the less present, but best to avoid entirely.
2. ***Identify Refined Grains and Fillers***: Look for "whole" as the first word in grain products. Avoid white flour, enriched flour, or products with a long ingredient list full of fillers and preservatives.
3. ***Examine Fats***: Avoid foods listing hydrogenated, partially hydrogenated, or palm oil, high in saturated fat. Focus on those using extra-virgin olive oil as the primary fat source.
4. ***Sodium Content***: Limit products with more than 200 mg of sodium per serving, as excess sodium can worsen liver inflammation and cardiovascular risk.
5. ***Artificial Additives***: Steer clear of artificial sweeteners, food colorings, and preservatives; choose products with a short, recognizable ingredient list.
6. ***Serving Size and Total Carbohydrates***: Verify the stated serving size and compare net carbohydrates (subtracting fiber) per serving. Prefer options with higher fiber and lower sugar.

7. ***"Low Fat" or "Diet" Food Traps***: These often compensate for taste by adding sugars or artificial flavors. Always check ingredients thoroughly.

Seasonal Produce Selection Guide for Optimal Nutrient Intake

Leveraging seasonal produce brings several advantages: fresher flavor, lower prices, superior nutrient density, and better environmental sustainability. For women managing fatty liver, seasonality also provides essential nutrient diversity to support metabolic and hormonal needs.

Spring/Summer Picks

- Leafy greens: Spinach, arugula, lettuce varieties
- Fresh herbs: Dill, basil, mint, parsley
- Cruciferous: Broccoli, cauliflower
- Tomatoes, zucchini, cucumbers, peppers
- Berries: Strawberries, raspberries, blueberries
- Stone fruits: Cherries, plums (use in moderation for sugar control)

Autumn/Winter Picks

- Root vegetables: Carrots, beets (watch portion for natural sugars)
- Squash: Butternut, acorn, pumpkin
- Brassicas: Brussels sprouts, cabbage, turnips, kale

- Citrus: Oranges, lemons, grapefruit (limit to one small portion per meal)
- Apples, pears (focus on green apple for lower sugar)

Year-Round Staples

- Onions, garlic (potent antioxidants)
- Celery, carrots (for soups, bases)
- Frozen berries or green vegetables (nutrient-dense off-season options)

When shopping, choose organic where possible for leafy greens and berries, which may have higher pesticide residues. Rotate selections every few weeks to gain a range of antioxidants and micronutrients.

Liver-Friendly Essentials Shopping List Builder

Constructing your essential shopping list each week ensures that your kitchen is always ready for meal prep without the stress of missing key ingredients. Use the template below and personalize with your preferred vegetables, proteins, and pantry needs:

Vegetables (choose 5–7 types):

- Spinach, kale, arugula, Swiss chard
- Broccoli, cauliflower, peppers
- Tomatoes, eggplant, zucchini
- Onions, garlic

Fruits (choose 2–3 types, focus on low sugar):

- Blueberries, strawberries, raspberries (fresh or frozen)
- Lemons, oranges, green apples
- Pomegranate seeds

Proteins:

- Skinless chicken breast, turkey breast
- Salmon, sardines, white fish filets
- Eggs
- Cans/jars of beans: chickpeas, lentils, black beans

Grains:

Rolled or steel-cut oats, quinoa, barley, brown rice

Dairy:

- Plain Greek yogurt (unsweetened)
- Feta, ricotta, or cottage cheese (reduced fat options)

Pantry:

- Olive oil (extra-virgin, first cold pressed)
- Raw, unsalted nuts (almonds, walnuts), seeds (pumpkin, sunflower, chia)
- Herbs and spices: Basil, thyme, oregano, cinnamon, cumin

Extras:

- Vinegar (balsamic, red wine)
- Canned tomatoes (plain)
- Low-sodium vegetable or chicken stock
- Lemons (for zest/juice), avocado, olives

When creating your list, match quantities to your weekly meal plan rotation and expected number of servings. A template posted on your fridge or kept as a digital note is helpful for ongoing efficiency.

Tips for Success: Keep the Most Used Items at the Front for Easy Access

Arrange your kitchen so that liver-safe, frequently used ingredients are easy to see and grab. Put vegetables at eye level, grains and legumes in clear containers, and snacks like nuts or yogurt at the front of your fridge. When an item runs low, immediately add it to your list for the next shop. This easy-access method nudges healthy habits and reduces the risk of defaulting to convenience or processed foods.

Carefully selecting and maintaining your liver-safe pantry, fridge, and freezer is one of the most powerful forms of self-care in your journey through a 21-day Mediterranean meal plan for fatty liver.

Remember: your environment shapes your habits. With a well-stocked kitchen anchored around antioxidant-rich produce, whole grains, lean proteins, and healthy fats and with a keen eye to seasonal variety and label details you ensure that every bite supports not only your liver, but also your overall metabolic, hormonal, and long-term health as a woman.

21-Day Grocery Lists and Shopping Maps (Role: Execution)

The core of a sustainable 21-day liver-friendly Mediterranean meal plan is smart grocery execution, thoughtful planning, strategic selection, and adaptive shopping that removes guesswork. For health-conscious women addressing fatty liver, consistency in grocery habits not only supports metabolic repair but also removes one of the biggest practical roadblocks: the uncertainty of what to buy, when, and where to find it. This chapter offers a detailed, actionable roadmap for executing your weekly shops with confidence, efficiency, and purpose.

Three Distinct Weekly Grocery Lists, Tailored to the Meal Plan Rotation

Reflecting the Mediterranean approach and the specific needs of women with fatty liver, each weekly grocery list is constructed to rotate core ingredients and prevent dietary monotony. This rotation supports nutrient diversity, helping to address unique female risk factors and hormonal fluctuations that influence liver fat accumulation and sensitivity to sugars.

Week 1: Foundation and Stabilizers

- ***Vegetables***: Spinach, kale, broccoli, zucchini, eggplant, red bell peppers, onions, garlic
- ***Fruits***: Blueberries, green apples, lemons
- ***Legumes***: Dried or canned chickpeas, lentils
- ***Whole Grains***: Rolled oats, quinoa, brown rice
- ***Protein***: Skinless chicken breast, salmon filets, eggs
- ***Dairy***: Plain Greek yogurt, feta cheese
- ***Healthy Fats***: Extra-virgin olive oil, raw almonds, walnuts
- ***Pantry***: Canned tomatoes (no added sugar/salt), balsamic vinegar, dried oregano, ground cumin

Week 2: Variety and Anti-Inflammatory Focus

- Vegetables: Swiss chard, arugula, cauliflower, Brussels sprouts, cherry tomatoes, mushrooms
- Fruits: Strawberries, oranges, pomegranate (seeded or juice, unsweetened, small quantity)
- Legumes: Black beans, cannellini beans
- Whole Grains: Farro, barley
- Protein: Turkey breast, sardines (packed in water or olive oil), eggs
- Dairy: Cottage cheese, ricotta
- Healthy Fats: Avocado, sunflower seeds, pumpkin seeds
- Pantry: Red wine vinegar, canned artichoke hearts, thyme, smoked paprika

Week 3: Seasonal and Nutrient-Rich Extensions

- ***Vegetables***: Broccoli rabe, leeks, butternut squash, beets (watch portion), sweet peppers, garlic (restock fresh)
- ***Fruits***: Raspberries, lemons, pears (focus on green/less sweet varieties)
- ***Legumes***: Split peas, mixed dried beans for soup
- ***Whole Grains***: Brown rice, barley, couscous (whole grain preferred)
- ***Protein***: White fish filets, skinless chicken thighs, eggs
- ***Dairy***: Reduced-fat goat cheese, plain yogurt
- ***Healthy Fats***: Olives, chia seeds, pumpkin seeds
- ***Pantry***: Low-salt vegetable broth, extra-virgin olive oil, basil, mint, parsley

Rotate these lists weekly to align meals with your plan's structure, accounting for household size and personal preferences. Use the previous chapter's inventory templates to review which items need replenishing after each week's shop.

Checklist for Prioritizing Fresh, Minimally Processed Items in Each Food Section

When navigating the grocery store, your selection process directly influences the effectiveness of a liver-friendly, low-sugar Mediterranean meal plan. Utilize these practical checklists for each section to keep choices clean, simple, and aligned with the dietary strategy:

Produce:

- ☐ Select vibrant, undamaged vegetables and fruits focus on seasonal and local for peak nutrition.
- ☐ Choose leafy greens and cruciferous vegetables frequently for their fiber and antioxidant content.
- ☐ Opt for organic on high-residue items if possible; wash thoroughly regardless.

Grains and Legumes:

- ☐ Shop the bulk bins or whole grain section; verify that labels list the single whole grain ingredient (e.g., "whole quinoa").
- ☐ Avoid packaged grain mixes with added flavors or sauces.
- ☐ Prefer low- or no-sodium canned legumes, or buy dried and batch-cook.

Proteins:

- ☐ Prioritize fresh, skinless poultry and fish rich in omega-3s (like salmon and sardines).
- ☐ Choose eggs with minimal processing cage-free or organic when possible.
- ☐ For plant-based, buy unseasoned legumes.

Dairy:

- ☐ Select plain Greek yogurt and reduced-fat cheeses, checking labels for added sugars or artificial stabilizers.
- ☐ Avoid flavored varieties ("fruit on the bottom," "vanilla," etc.) due to hidden sugar.

Healthy Fats, Nuts, and Seeds:

- ☐ Seek out raw, unsalted nuts and seeds.
- ☐ Buy extra-virgin olive oil in dark bottles for freshness.
- ☐ Limit processed spreads and flavored oils.

Pantry and Herbs:

- ☐ Prefer canned tomatoes, beans, and artichoke hearts labeled "no added sugar" and "no/lower salt."
- ☐ Shop for fresh or dried herbs and spices over pre-mixed seasoning blends, which often contain sodium or preservatives.

Strategies for Shopping Within Time and Budget Constraints

A common barrier to maintaining liver-friendly eating is the perceived expense and time required for shopping. Apply the following strategies to overcome these hurdles:

- Prioritize core ingredients (leafy greens, beans, whole grains, eggs, olive oil) as budget-friendly staples. These can form the bulk of meals and keep costs low.
- Shop perimeter aisles first, where fresh produce, meats, and dairy are found. Interior aisles should mainly be visited for pantry essentials.
- Plan your shop around weekly store sales circulars; base some produce and proteins on discounts and in-season specials.
- Buy larger packs and batch-cook grains, legumes, and proteins, freezing portions to reduce both prep time and mid-week shopping.
- Choose frozen vegetables and fruits as backups—they retain nutrients and can be less costly when out of season.
- Limit specialty or imported items to once or twice monthly; the bulk of Mediterranean, liver-friendly ingredients are basic and widely available.
- For time, make a focused list matching your weekly meal plan and shop during off-peak grocery hours (early mornings, late evenings, or weekday afternoons).

If managing a very tight budget, prioritize plant-based proteins and legumes (chickpeas, lentils, beans), buy whole grains in bulk, and focus on versatile vegetables like cabbage, carrots, and greens. Minimize convenience meals and individually packaged snacks, which tend to cost more and include less liver-friendly ingredients.

Grocery Store Mapping Tool for Efficient Navigation and Limiting Impulse Buys

Mapping your route through the store is essential to save time and stick to your liver-friendly plan. This reduces not only distraction and fatigue, but also the odds of impulse purchases that undermine dietary goals. Use this simple mapping approach:

1. ***Start in produce***: Begin with your fruit and vegetable list, loading up on the bulk of your food for the week at the start—fill half your cart with produce first.
2. ***Proceed to proteins***: Move next to the meat/fish department for poultry, fish, and eggs.
3. ***Dairy case***: Select only what is on your list (plain yogurt, cheese) and skip dessert and processed dairy aisles.
4. ***Grains and legumes***: Head to the bulk foods section or natural foods aisle for oats, barley, quinoa, beans, and lentils.
5. ***Pantry staples***: Visit the canned goods section for no-sugar-added tomatoes and beans, bypassing processed sauces, soups, and meal kits.
6. ***Healthy fats and snacks***: Go to the oils/nuts/seeds aisle, again sticking to your list.

7. Finish with herbs, spices, and specialty items for flavor.

Additional tips:

- Stick to the outer perimeter; avoid wandering through snack/candy or heavily processed food aisles.
- Keep a printed list with checkboxes for each section; only allow yourself to add off-list items if they're true liver-friendly basics on sale.
- Use a separate "never" list to remind yourself of foods that are off-plan (white breads, sugary cereals, processed deli meats, flavored yogurts, etc.).
- If shopping with family or children, delegate list-based tasks to keep the trip efficient and focused.

This approach helps maintain a rapid, deliberate pace that discourages impulse buys and supports your health goals every step of the way.

Troubleshooting Guide for Managing Substitutions Due to In-Store Shortages

Despite the best plans, ingredient shortages are a reality. Flexibility, without sacrificing dietary integrity, is crucial for staying on track with your 21-day meal plan. Follow these guidelines for smart substitutions:

Vegetables:

- Substitute different greens (e.g., replace kale with spinach or Swiss chard).
- Use frozen mixed vegetables if fresh options are unavailable—they're nutritious and often more affordable.
- Swap within color/texture profiles: If bell peppers are out, try zucchini or eggplant.

Fruits:

- Aim for low-sugar varieties. Berries are interchangeable; if strawberries are out, use blueberries or raspberries.
- If citrus is absent, use green apples or pomegranate for brightness and antioxidants.

Legumes:

Swap among beans and lentils freely—almost any can be interchanged in stews, salads, and soups without changing the nutritional goal.

Whole Grains:

If quinoa is unavailable, try barley, farro, or even brown rice. Use oats in place of other grains for breakfast recipes.

Proteins:

- Replace fish varieties with another lean fish or plant-based protein (like beans or lentils).
- Use eggs in place of poultry for a meal in a pinch.

Dairy:

- Switch among plain Greek yogurt, cottage cheese, or ricotta—just watch for label sugar content.
- Substitute with unsweetened plant-based yogurts sparingly, if dairy is out.

Nuts, Seeds, and Healthy Fats:

- Substitute among raw, unsalted nuts and seeds (almonds, walnuts, sunflower, pumpkin, chia, etc.).
- If extra-virgin olive oil is low, use small amounts of avocado oil for cooking.

Herbs and Spices:

- *Flexible*: While certain combinations are classic, swap basil for parsley, or dill for mint, depending on season and store supply.
- Dried herbs are a backup if you can't find them fresh.

Always reference your ingredient inventory from Chapter 5 before shopping. Sometimes you already have a suitable replacement at home. Update your meal plan after each shop as needed to reflect what's available, ensuring your

Mediterranean strategy remains intact, and your meals remain liver-friendly

Master grocery list rotation, prioritize fresh and minimally processed options, shop strategically, map your store route, and troubleshoot ingredient gaps with confidence to remove obstacles to success on the 21-day liver-friendly Mediterranean plan. Each week, these practices stabilize your routine, save time and money, and empower you to make every meal a step toward better liver and overall health, especially for women whose needs are uniquely nuanced through every phase of life.

Simple Meal Prep and Batch Cooking Strategies (Role: Application)

As you move from strategic grocery shopping to the heart of daily action, efficient meal prep becomes your most practical tool for sustaining a low-sugar Mediterranean meal plan tailored for fatty liver health. The principles you've learned so far prioritizing fresh, unprocessed foods, choosing lean proteins, emphasizing fiber-packed grains and legumes come alive in your kitchen through simple, repeatable routines. This chapter is designed to close the gap between your ideal grocery list and what actually appears on your plate, streamlining the journey from ingredients to satisfying, liver-supportive meals.

Meal prep not only saves time but also reduces daily stress and minimizes food waste—it is particularly important for women managing fatty liver, whose metabolic needs often demand regularity, nutrient density, and portion control. When prep is systematized, it becomes easier to avoid hidden sugars, accidental over-portioning, and the lure of convenience foods that can disrupt liver recovery and metabolic balance.

Meal Prep Sessions Scheduled for Optimal Freshness and Minimal Waste

Strategic meal prep requires scheduling focused sessions that align with ingredient shelf life and your weekly meal rotation. Begin by reviewing your weekly Mediterranean meal plan and grocery inventory. Designate prep times directly after your main grocery shop. For most, two sessions per week are ideal: one major session immediately after shopping, and a shorter mid-week session for refreshing produce, prepping quick-cook proteins, and adjusting as needed.

Why schedule two sessions? As much as batch-prepping everything at once seems efficient, certain liver-friendly ingredients—like leafy greens, ripe fruits, and some seafood—lose flavor and nutrition if stored too long. **Splitting your routine allows you to:**

- Wash, chop, and store sturdy vegetables (e.g., carrots, cruciferous veg, onions, and peppers) and initial proteins (chicken, legumes) immediately.
- Cook and portion grains or legumes that will be used throughout the week.
- Portion fresh leafy greens, berries, and delicate produce in the second session to maximize crispness and flavor.

- Review what's left mid-week, which helps avoid waste and enables a quick pivot if plans change or an ingredient runs low.

Here is a practical approach to scheduling your meal prep:

1. **Major Prep (Shopping Day):**
    - Wash and dry sturdy produce.
    - Batch-cook proteins (chicken, eggs, fish if using within 2 days), grains (brown rice, quinoa, barley), and legumes.
    - Portion or roast vegetables that will maintain quality for several days.
    - Prepare dressings or marinated proteins.
2. **Mini Refresh (Mid-Week):**
    - Wash and store delicate greens and herbs.
    - Prepare hard-boiled eggs or quick fish for the next 2-3 meals.
    - Store cut fruits or make a simple fruit compote for snacks and breakfasts.

Adopting this rhythm allows daily meals to almost assemble themselves. This approach is especially valuable for women who are balancing multiple priorities and need consistent energy, digestion, and metabolic support.

Batch Cooking Plans for Proteins, Grains, and Vegetables

Batch cooking is the backbone of your 21-day liver-friendly Mediterranean plan. By preparing core components in volume, you create flexible building blocks for the week, making it far easier to stick to your liver-supportive goals, even on the busiest days.

Proteins:

- ***Chicken/Turkey***: Roast or poach skinless breasts, thighs, or cutlets in portions large enough for two to three meals. Shred or cube and store in airtight containers. Use for salads, wraps, or mixed grain bowls.
- ***Fish***: Bake or grill fillets (salmon, white fish, sardines) for up to two days' worth of meals; avoid prepping more than you'll eat in 48 hours to keep flavor and nutrition intact.
- ***Eggs***: Hard-boil a dozen eggs at a time. These make for quick breakfasts, snacks, or an easy protein upgrade to salads.
- ***Legumes***: Cook a pot of chickpeas, lentils, or beans—these last up to a week when properly stored and are extremely versatile.

Grains:

- Prepare large batches of brown rice, farro, barley, or quinoa. Cool completely, portion, and refrigerate for up to five days.
- Consider pre-portioning individual containers for grab-and-go lunches or breakfasts (e.g., overnight oats, grain bowls with fruit and nuts).

Vegetables:

- Roast or steam a sheet tray of hardy vegetables (broccoli, cauliflower, squash, sweet potatoes, carrots). These reheat well and retain texture for days.
- Prep raw salad bases: Spinach, kale, or mixed greens wash and keep best when spun dry and loosely stored in lined containers.
- Chop bell peppers, cucumbers, radishes, and carrots in advance for snacks or quick salads.

Each batch is a modular element; combine as needed with sauce, a squeeze of fresh citrus, and a handful of herbs to create low-sugar, Mediterranean-inspired meals in minutes. This approach supports nutrient-dense, minimally processed eating, which is central to liver health.

Storage Systems to Maximize Nutrient Retention and Food Safety

Proper storage isn't just about keeping food edible, it's essential for maintaining maximum nutrient density, preserving flavor, and ensuring food safety. This is particularly critical in a liver-supportive meal plan; lean proteins and vegetables can quickly lose quality, while improper storage increases the risk of spoilage and foodborne illness.

Key Storage Guidelines:

- ***Glass and Steel Containers***: Favor non-reactive, BPA-free containers. Glass is ideal for grains, cooked proteins, and roasted vegetables. It does not absorb odors and allows for easy reheating in the oven or microwave.
- ***Airtight Jars for Dressings and Sauces***: Prevent oxidation and loss of delicate flavors in vinaigrettes and homemade marinades.
- ***Produce Bags and Crisper Drawers***: Use designated produce bags to manage airflow and moisture for leafy greens and herbs. Hardier produce can be stored in the crisper with a slightly damp paper towel.
- ***Refrigeration Timelines***:
    - Cooked proteins: 2–4 days (fish at the lower end, eggs and chicken slightly longer)
    - Cooked grains and legumes: Up to 5 days

    - Roasted or steamed vegetables: 3–4 days for best flavor and texture
    - Raw chopped veg for snacking: 4–5 days, depending on the initial freshness
- ***Label Everything***: Add prep dates to containers—a small but vital step for tracking food safety and minimizing accidental waste.

Nutrient Retention Tips:

- Store cut fruits and vegetables in airtight containers to slow nutrient loss from air exposure.
- Keep citrus separate until ready to use, as citrus juices can speed up the breakdown of greens and some proteins.
- Don't pre-cut avocados; wait until serving to slice for salads or bowls, to avoid browning and loss of antioxidants.

By implementing this method, you extend the shelf life and nutritional value of your meal components, keep flavors vibrant, and reduce the temptation to grab nutritionally empty packaged snacks.

Freezer-friendly recipe adaptations for busy weeks

Freezer prep is an invaluable add-on for those weeks when schedules are unpredictable or motivation dips. Many

Mediterranean, liver-friendly dishes adapt beautifully to freezing without sacrificing taste or health benefits, provided you follow a few basic rules:

- ***Soups and Stews***: Lentil, bean, and vegetable stews freeze exceptionally well. Portion individual servings into freezer-safe containers, leaving some headspace for expansion.
- ***Batch-Cooked Grains and Legumes***: Cooked brown rice, quinoa, beans, and lentils can be portioned and frozen in zip-top bags or small containers. Lay bags flat for quick thawing.
- ***Roasted Vegetable Mixes***: While some leafy or watery vegetables lose texture, roasted carrots, squash, cauliflower, and peppers thaw and reheat well for sides or lunch bowls.
- ***Lean Protein Patties***: Turkey or chicken patties can be pre-cooked and frozen; just thaw and reheat in the oven or pan.
- ***Egg Muffins/Omelettes***: Bake a batch of vegetable-egg muffins in muffin tins, then freeze; they are ready for a quick breakfast or snack.

Tips for Effective Freezer Use:

- Cool foods completely before freezing to prevent freezer burn and textural decline.
- Use small, clearly labeled containers for easy portion control.

- Thaw overnight in the fridge for best texture, or in the microwave using the defrost setting.
- For optimal quality, consume freezer meals within 2–3 months.

Freezer meals are not only convenient for last-minute dinners or rushed mornings; they are also a safeguard against falling back on processed or high-sugar convenience foods when time is tight. With a few hours of prep, you buffer yourself against common barriers that derail healthy eating and liver repair.

Weekly Meal Prep Task Planner

Consistent results stem from a simple, reusable task planner that tracks prepping, cooking, storage, and menu assembly for each week of your 21-day plan. Here's a sample outline to guide your sessions:

Pre-Prep (Review and Inventory):

- Review the coming week's meal plan.
- Cross-check pantry and fridge against your ingredient inventory (see Chapter 5).
- Make a prep day schedule blocking out 1-2 hour slots.

Major Prep (Shopping Day or Night):

- Wash and chop all sturdy vegetables and some fruit.
- Start a batch of brown rice, barley, or quinoa.
- Preheat the oven for roasting veg and proteins.

- Boil eggs; cook beans or lentils if using dried.
- Prepare a marinade or quick dressing.

Assembly Line:

- Portion proteins into serving-size containers.
- Divide grains into ready-to-grab batches.
- Mix raw salad bases for the first half of the week.
- Decant snacks (nuts, chopped veggies) into containers.

Mid-Week Refresh:

- Wash delicate greens and herbs.
- Prep remaining proteins and fruit.
- Check for anything nearing expiry and plan meals to use them.

Storage and Tracking:

- Label all containers with dates and dish names.
- Place snacks and grab-and-go items at front of the fridge for easy access.
- Update your tracking chart (see Chapter 8) to reflect prepped meals and portions.

Establish these steps and repeat them to transform meal planning from daily chores into a streamlined weekly routine one that promotes liver repair, maintains steady energy and blood sugar, and guarantees variety and enjoyment in every meal.

Efficiency in the kitchen is foundational for women seeking sustainable progress in reversing or managing fatty liver. Through deliberate meal prep scheduling, batch cooking, smart storage systems, freezer-friendly adaptations, and a weekly task planner, you build a meal routine that protects liver function, curbs added sugar, and reduces stress.

These strategies turn your intentions into action, bringing Mediterranean wellness not just to the pantry, but to every bite you eat. By developing these habits over your 21-day journey and beyond you invest in a system that fits real life, preserves nutritional integrity, and supports lasting liver health.

Tracking Meals, Progress, and Symptoms (Role: Measurement)

Building a lasting liver-friendly routine goes far beyond just preparing healthy meals; it also requires clear self-monitoring and honest feedback. Consistent tracking not only provides crucial motivation, but it helps you see patterns, recognize what's working, and advocate for adjustments tailored to women's unique metabolic challenges in managing fatty liver. In this chapter, you'll learn how to keep a detailed record of meals, sugar intake, progress, and key liver health symptoms during your 21-day Mediterranean plan for optimal insight and accountability.

Daily Meal and Sugar Intake Log Designed for Mediterranean Liver Plans

A primary driver of liver health improvement is what you put on your plate, meal by meal, day after day. For women managing fatty liver, tracking what you eat particularly your intake of added and naturally occurring sugars is non-negotiable. Even meals full of whole foods may contain "hidden" sugar sources that easily add up and sabotage hard-earned metabolic gains. The foundation of your tracking system should be a daily log that captures every meal and snack, with an explicit column for sugar content.

To design a daily log suited for a low-sugar Mediterranean lifestyle, include these essential fields:

- Date and Day (to analyze trends over weeks)
- Meal/Time (breakfast, lunch, dinner, snack, and their timing)
- Foods Eaten (breakdown by main dish, sides, beverages, and condiments)
- Portion Sizes (using visual cues or measurements)
- Estimated or Labeled Sugar Content (total grams for the meal/snack)
- Notes on Preparation (cooked at home, prepped in advance, eaten out, etc.)
- Satiety Rating (e.g., 1 = still hungry, 5 = comfortably full)

Before you sit down to eat, jot down your planned meal; after eating, reflect on the actual foods and any modifications or additions. For sugar tracking, check nutrition labels for packaged items, use online tools for common produce or grains, and reference your meal plan's recipe chart, especially for Mediterranean dishes featuring occasional fruit, yogurt, or sauces. Remember, even a drizzle of honey or balsamic glaze should be logged.

For best results, keep your log visible in your kitchen, or use a notes app on your phone for on-the-go tracking. The act of logging alone increases mindfulness, helping prevent unintentional deviations from the meal plan and ensuring you keep overall sugar intake consistently low—essential for turning liver-friendly intentions into results.

Self-Monitoring Symptom Checklist, Including Key Markers for Women

Fatty liver often develops and progresses quietly, but several early signs and physical cues can be tracked at home—especially relevant for women, who may experience subtle symptoms linked to hormonal cycles or metabolic differences. A robust symptom checklist supercharges your awareness and offers early warning if extra support or plan adjustments are needed.

Your symptom checklist should be completed daily or every other day. Include the following markers:

- ***Energy Levels (Morning and Afternoon)***: Are you fatigued even after sleep? Do you experience an energy drop in the late morning or afternoon?
- ***Mood and Mental Clarity***: Any new or unexplained irritability, anxiety, or "brain fog?"
- ***Digestive Comfort***: Noting bloating, fullness after moderate meals, or unpredictable bowel changes.

- ***Visible Abdominal Changes***: Is your waist measurement increasing or do you notice extra fullness, especially in the upper right abdomen?
- ***Skin and Eyes***: Check for any yellowing or unusual rashes.
- ***Sleep Quality***: Difficulties falling or staying asleep, especially if previously uncommon.
- ***Joint or Muscle Pain***: Any new aches or pains, as inflammation is sometimes an associated factor.
- ***Menstrual Cycle Changes (for pre-menopausal women)***: Document irregularities, increased PMS symptoms, or cycle changes.

For each marker, use simple scales (such as 1–5 for severity or "yes/no" for presence/absence). Brief daily notes can provide context e.g., "minor bloating after lunch, resolved by evening." Over time, these patterns inform whether dietary changes are lessening symptoms or if new issues are appearing.

Women in particular should watch for subtle variability tied to hormonal cycles, as research suggests unique hormonal and metabolic patterns influence both risk and progression of fatty liver disease. Tracking these alongside diet helps distinguish what a dietary response is and what may be influenced by other life factors.

Weekly Progress Dashboard Template for Tracking Energy, Mood, and Bloating

To see big-picture changes, it's vital to pull daily details together into a weekly dashboard—your "at-a-glance" health index. This summary not only drives motivation but also flags trends quickly, guiding timely tweaks to your Mediterranean liver plan.

Set up a simple template either in a notebook, spreadsheet, or printable chart. For each week, create rows for:

- Average Daily Energy (morning/afternoon, scored from your daily logs)
- Average Mood Rating (pull data from your checklist; note peaks and valleys)
- Number of Days with Bloating or Digestive Upset
- Average Sleep Quality (hours and subjective rating)
- Number of Days Plan Was Fully Followed (meals and snacks)
- Notable Symptoms or Trends (brief summary—e.g., "Steady energy, but mild bloating after dinner")

Populate your dashboard at the end of each week, reviewing not only numbers but written notes for deeper patterns. For example, a week with high adherence but increased bloating might suggest a specific ingredient isn't tolerated, or that meal timing needs review.

Use the dashboard as a feedback mirror: Is fatigue dropping as sugar intake falls? Is digestive comfort built with more fiber-rich legumes and vegetables? Are mood swings stabilizing? This visual comparison accelerates your learning curve and supports sustainable change.

Criteria for Evaluating Meal Plan Adherence Versus Clinical Outcome Signals

While the act of recording daily inputs is valuable, it is equally important to set clear benchmarks for assessing adherence and evaluating whether your efforts are driving meaningful improvement in liver and metabolic health. This involves separating process goals (e.g., how closely you followed the meal plan) from outcome signals (actual changes in symptoms, energy, or measurements).

To evaluate adherence, use these criteria:

- Number of Days in the Week All Meals Matched Plan Guidelines (lean protein, low sugar, Mediterranean focus)
- Portion Control Achieved (measured by whether all servings align with plan recommendations)
- Added Sugar Intake at or Below Plan Maximum (verify with your log for the week)
- Frequency of Eating Out or Deviations from Home-Prepared Meals

For outcome signals, focus on clinical and functional improvements, such as:

- Reduction in Bloating, Abdominal Fullness, or Discomfort
- Stable or Improved Energy and Mood (as shown on your dashboard)
- Waist Circumference Changes (measured weekly—modest reductions are encouraging)
- Improvements in Sleep or Mental Clarity (from your log)
- Fewer Sugar Cravings or Less Afternoon Fatigue

When adherence is high but outcome improvement is lacking, review your meal choices for hidden sugars or excess portions, and ensure your symptom checklist captures everything relevant. On the other hand, positive clinical signals with moderate adherence might indicate your body is particularly responsive to even partial dietary changes.

For women, hormonal fluctuations may add complexity to this evaluation. Track your menstrual cycle alongside the above data to contextualize short-term changes, and be prepared to seek clinical input if symptoms persist or worsen despite strong adherence.

21-Day Tracking and Feedback Chart for Printable or Digital Use

The backbone of this self-monitoring system is a 21-day comprehensive tracking chart. This tool organizes both your food choices and your physical responses, making tangible the invisible progress that often comes with Mediterranean, liver-supportive eating.

Your chart should contain these columns for each day:

1. Date and Day
2. Meal/Snack Entry (with time)
3. Food/Drink Consumed (detailed)
4. Sugar Content Estimate (grams per meal/snack)
5. Total Daily Sugar Intake
6. Water Intake (glasses)
7. Satiety Rating (after each meal)
8. Key Symptom Ratings (energy, mood, bloating, sleep quality, digestive comfort)
9. Notes (hunger levels, cravings, menstrual status, lifestyle factors)

At the end of each week, use the dashboard template to transfer your summary data. This process facilitates weekly "mini-reflections"—adjusting next week's meal prep, targeting specific symptoms, or celebrating improvements.

A digital spreadsheet (using basic formulas to sum daily sugar intake and auto-average symptom/rating data) works well for many, while a printed chart posted in your kitchen supports daily accountability. Both formats ensure the core goal: making consistent, positive actions visible and measurable.

Key tips for maximizing your tracking:

- Record entries immediately rather than waiting until the end of the day
- Be honest about deviations documenting "off-plan" moments is equally valuable
- Correlate symptoms with specific meals (trouble after a particular dinner? Note it!)
- Share your chart with a supportive friend or healthcare provider if extra motivation or insight is needed

Integrating Tracking into Your 21-Day Mediterranean Liver Plan

Adhering to a Mediterranean, low-sugar liver plan is a commitment particularly for women balancing career, family, and health priorities. But research confirms that systematic tracking is one of the most effective drivers of sustained dietary change. The more data you collect, the faster you'll learn what works for your unique body and circumstances.

For best results, consider setting a 2-minute reminder after each meal to complete your log. Pair tracking with an enjoyable ritual (like sipping herbal tea or listening to music) to make it more rewarding, not a chore. Over your 21 days, you'll have a clear narrative of how Mediterranean eating, meal structure, and sugar reduction work together— and how your personal signals are evolving.

Tracking doesn't just confirm what you already know; it surfaces hidden obstacles, provides reality checks during plateaus, and highlights "small wins" that add up to real change, especially for women, whose fatty liver progression and remission may not mirror men's in visibility or timeline.

The measurement strategies described in this chapter are your compass for the 21-day journey and beyond. By maintaining a robust daily meal and sugar intake log, self-monitoring your key symptoms, and leveraging weekly dashboards and the full 21-day feedback chart, you anchor your Mediterranean liver plan in the realities of your day-to-day life. This measurement system transforms dietary intention into meaningful, trackable action protecting your liver, elevating your energy, and clarifying the path to sustainable improvement.

The next and final practical layer is learning to interpret your records when to troubleshoot setbacks, when to celebrate progress, and when to adjust strategies for lasting change. As you embark on the final phase of your journey, your tracking charts will become not just a record, but a springboard to lifelong liver health and Mediterranean vitality.

Adjusting and Sustaining Your Liver-Friendly Routine (Role: Troubleshooting)

As you move through the 21-day liver-friendly Mediterranean meal plan, the journey doesn't end with the completion of the initial cycle. The true success lies in your ability to adapt, troubleshoot barriers, and sustain these healthy habits for long-term liver wellness. This chapter brings together practical strategies to help you modify your plan when facing obstacles, confidently navigate challenging social settings, recognize when professional input is needed, and extend your Mediterranean habits seamlessly beyond the first 21 days.

Rules-of-Thumb for Modifying Menu Items and Ingredients

Fatty liver improvement is rarely linear, especially for women. Changes in metabolism, hormones, or life circumstances can influence not only your meal preferences but also your body's response to specific ingredients or patterns. Rather than viewing the meal plan as rigid, think of it as a customizable framework. When you notice slow progress or run into setbacks, use these rules-of-thumb to recalibrate while preserving the plan's liver-friendly foundation:

1. ***Swap, Don't Skip***. If a recipe calls for a vegetable or protein you don't tolerate or have on hand (e.g., tomatoes or chickpeas), simply swap in another Mediterranean-approved option from your pantry list. Cauliflower, lentils, or leafy greens are excellent substitutes that maintain the nutritional profile.
2. ***Downshift Sugar, Always***. Whether you're baking, preparing sauces, or choosing snacks, reduce or eliminate added sugars. Opt for spices like cinnamon, vanilla, or citrus zest for flavor. Replace sweetened yogurts with plain Greek yogurt topped with berries or nuts, and use fresh fruit sparingly as a sweet accent, not a main dish.
3. ***Choose Whole Over Processed***. If you're short on time, resist the temptation of processed, convenience foods promising "healthy" or "low-fat" benefits. Most processed foods contain hidden sugars and unhealthy fats. Instead, lean on batch-cooked grains, lean proteins (like grilled chicken or beans), and washed, chopped produce for quick assembly.
4. ***Go for Olive Oil, Not Butter***. Keep extra-virgin olive oil as your default fat source for dressings, sautéing, and baking. Replace any recipe's butter or cream with

olive oil or Greek yogurt to reduce saturated fat intake and support liver repair.

5. ***Manage Portions Mindfully***. If your energy plateaus or digestion feels heavy, try using smaller plates, focusing on mostly vegetables and lean protein, and saving richer items—like cheese or starchy sides—for occasional, smaller servings.
6. ***Batch and Freeze***. Encountering a busy week? Double Mediterranean stew, bean soup, or roasted vegetable recipes and freeze portions for fast, on-plan meals later. This prevents resorting to convenience foods and helps maintain consistent nutrition.
7. ***Hydrate, Hydrate, Hydrate***. If an unexpected craving or fatigue appears, try increasing your water intake before modifying meals. In many cases, dehydration amplifies hunger and sluggishness—common issues among women with fatty liver.

Navigational Checklist for Challenging Situations: Social Events, Dining Out, and Travel

Social events, restaurant meals, and travel periods are notorious for disrupting healthy routines. However, with advance planning and a toolkit of strategies, you can protect your progress and enjoy connection without derailing your liver-friendly habits.

Before the Event or Trip:

- Review the menu or ask your host about available options. Identify dishes that feature lean proteins (fish, chicken, legumes), vegetables, and olive oil, and plan to decline high-sugar or battered items.
- Offer to bring a Mediterranean-approved dish, such as a colorful bean salad with lemon-olive oil dressing or a fruit-and-nut platter.
- Eat a small, balanced meal or snack at home (such as hummus with veggies, or a boiled egg with greens) to reduce hunger-driven, off-plan choices at the event.
- Pack portable options for travel: unsalted nuts, whole fruit, and homemade wraps with lean protein and greens travel well and keep you within your meal plan.

<u>During the Event:</u>

- Prioritize vegetables and legumes choose salads with vinaigrette (dressing on the side), grilled vegetables, or vegetable-based soups.
- Choose grilled, baked, or steamed proteins, avoiding fried or breaded selections, high-fat cuts, or sugary sauces.
- Watch portions of bread, rice, or pasta. If offered, ask for a vegetable or legume substitute or a half-portion.
- Decline or limit alcohol, opting for sparkling water with citrus or unsweetened herbal tea.

After the Event:

- Log what you ate and how you feel. Acknowledge any deviations without judgment, and focus on resuming your standard routine at your very next meal.
- Use your tracking chart to identify triggers (e.g., hunger before parties, peer pressure to eat dessert) and plan better strategies for the next occasion.

Signals Indicating the Need for Recalibration or Professional Input

Self-monitoring is your first line of feedback, but some signals mean it's time to pause and assess whether adjustments or a clinician's guidance are needed. Keep an eye out for these flags:

- ***Persistent fatigue***, severe digestive discomfort, or unexplained symptoms lasting more than two weeks despite full adherence to the plan.
- ***Plateau in energy or mood***, increasing abdominal fullness, or no improvement in liver health markers (as discussed with your healthcare provider).
- ***Consistent inability to follow the meal plan*** due to cravings, hunger, or life disruptions—these may signal undiagnosed nutrient deficiencies or hormonal imbalances, especially prevalent in women.
- ***Significant changes in weight*** (rapid loss or gain), jaundice (yellowing of skin or eyes), or persistent bloating/swelling.

- ***Menstrual irregularities or significant increase in PMS symptoms***, which may signal metabolic stress in pre-menopausal women.

If any of these situations occur, bring your meal and symptom logs to your healthcare professional for review. Dieticians can help recalibrate your Mediterranean meal plan, adjust portions, or identify foods that may be interfering with progress. Your logs provide an invaluable "baseline" for more personalized advice.

Maintenance Plan Framework: Avoiding Recipe Fatigue After 21 Days

Once you've built momentum through your 21-day plan, it's common to worry about running out of meal ideas or reverting to old habits. The secret to sustainability is balancing routine with variety, using a flexible framework that encourages experimentation within safe boundaries:

- ***Rotate Proteins and Base Recipes***. Alternate between fish, chicken, legumes, tofu, and eggs for main dishes. Use the meal builder templates from earlier chapters to swap in different vegetables, whole grains, herbs, and spices weekly.
- ***Explore Global Mediterranean Flavors***. Branch out by exploring North African, Middle Eastern, or Southern European adaptations—think Moroccan chickpea stew, Greek lentil soup, or Spanish gazpacho.

These variations use the same core liver-friendly ingredients.

- ***Batch Prepare Versatile Components***. Cook a pot of whole grains, roast extra vegetables, or prepare a double batch of a favorite sauce. Store these in the fridge for easy assembly into different meals throughout the week.
- ***Simplify Shopping with Theme Weeks***. Each week, pick a "theme" e.g., Italian, Provençal, or Levantine and plan your menu around it. This provides variety and helps streamline shopping for herbs, spices, and centerpiece ingredients.
- ***Schedule Mini-Refreshes***. Every two to four weeks, review your logs and symptom trends. Celebrate what's working, and swap out one or two recipes that feel tired for something fresh from your Mediterranean recipe index or reputable liver health resources.
- ***Keep Snacks Fresh and Simple***. Prepare rotating snack options like cucumber slices with hummus, roasted chickpeas, or plain Greek yogurt with a pinch of cinnamon and nuts. These snacks curb hunger and boost variety without extra sugar.

By viewing your meal plan as living and evolving, you'll guard against palate fatigue and strengthen your commitment to liver wellness with an ever-adapting Mediterranean toolkit.

Personalized Habit Adjustment Worksheet

Successful adjustment begins with structured reflection and planning. The worksheet below serves as a built-in troubleshooting and growth tool; use it monthly, or whenever you feel routine slipping or results plateauing.

Personalized Habit Adjustment Worksheet:

1. **Reflection (Last 2 weeks)**
    - Which meals or snacks consistently support my energy and comfort?
    - What was my biggest challenge or deviation, and what triggered it?
2. **Analysis**
    - Are there common ingredients or recipes that don't leave me satisfied?
    - Did I encounter new symptoms or persistent cravings?
    - How did social events, travel, or stress influence my choices?
3. **Action Planning**
    - What 1-2 recipes or meal patterns need a refresh? Which options am I excited to try from my recipe list?
    - Which strategies will I use for my most likely challenge next week (e.g., prepping snacks, planning social eating)?

- How will I reward myself for consistency (non-food rewards like a new cookbook, time outdoors, or mindfulness activity)?

4. **Track, Review, Adjust**
   - Commit to tracking symptoms, energy, and meal satisfaction for the next 7–14 days.
   - Set a follow-up date to review, using your dashboard, and adjust again as needed.

This worksheet is designed to be revisited regularly. The answers become your playbook for evolving your Mediterranean liver plan, supporting ongoing personalization and preventing boredom or burnout.

Empowering your liver-friendly routine doesn't mean fighting for perfection or fearing setbacks. As women with or at risk for fatty liver, your progress can ebb and flow with life's rhythms, hormonal changes, and daily unpredictability. The Mediterranean principles, especially when tailored to be low in sugar and rich in protective plant foods, offer the nutritional versatility to weather such changes gracefully.

Keep your troubleshooting tools visible and reflect regularly using structured worksheets. This approach transforms each obstacle into a learning opportunity, each plateau into a prompt for gentle adjustment, and each success into fuel for long-term change. The core skills ingredient swaps, portion mindfulness, batch prep, and honest meal logs remain powerful assets that support you well beyond the initial 21 days.

In your journey to lasting liver health, these troubleshooting and maintenance techniques are the difference-makers transforming a static diet into a dynamic, enjoyable lifestyle rooted in resilience, pleasure, and self-compassion. With each adjustment, you're not merely maintaining your progress you're building an ever-stronger foundation for lifelong liver vitality.

Conclusion

Completing a focused 21-day liver-friendly Mediterranean plan is a significant achievement, but the real power lies in transitioning these foundations into lasting daily habits. To sustain your momentum, carry forward the meal structures, tracking charts, and flexible recipe templates you've learned, but adapt them to suit changes in routine and personal taste. Start each week by reviewing your grocery inventory, selecting a handful of favorite Mediterranean core recipes, and batch prepping a few essentials like cooked grains, roasted vegetables, and portions of lean protein or legumes. This investment on your day off streamlines weekday choices and minimizes fallback on processed or high-sugar options.

Continue using your daily meal and symptom log as a practical accountability tool. Tracking doesn't need to be exhaustive; simply noting meal composition, portion sizes, and any fluctuations in energy or digestive comfort helps reveal trends and flag recipes or habits that consistently work for you. Every few weeks, reflect on your logs to celebrate victories and identify small, actionable tweaks. This ongoing feedback loop enables you to evolve the plan with less effort while maintaining its liver-friendly core.

Listen to your body, and empower yourself to act decisively if challenges arise during transitions. While minor fluctuations are normal as you adapt to a maintenance routine, there are clear indicators that signal a need for professional guidance. If you experience persistent fatigue, lasting digestive upset, or symptoms like jaundice or pronounced, unexplained bloating despite adhering to your meal patterns, consult your healthcare provider promptly.

Rapid changes in weight or the return of pre-diet symptoms especially for women who may notice menstrual irregularities or worsening premenstrual symptoms due to metabolic stress are also flags to review your logs and seek tailored medical advice. Be proactive in sharing your meal and symptom records, as these offer important context for more effective adjustments.

For most women, the sustainability of a liver-friendly diet hinges on variety and the practical ease of meal planning. The low-sugar Mediterranean framework supports both, emphasizing abundant vegetables, legumes, whole grains, fish, poultry, and generous use of olive oil, while minimizing added sugars and processed foods. The flexibility to rotate produce and protein such as alternating between lentil salads, fish stews, and bean-based soups prevents taste fatigue and ensures broad nutrient coverage. Spices and fresh herbs add interest without relying on sugar, and simple snack options like nuts, yogurt, or crudités make healthy choices the default, not the exception.

Over time, this approach becomes a sustainable protector for liver health. Mediterranean patterns, when adapted to limit sugar and saturated fat, help improve liver enzyme profiles and support metabolic wellness, particularly for women whose risks are influenced by hormonal and life-stage factors. By prioritizing plant foods and heart-healthy fats, and using food logs to personalize the journey, you create a resilient routine that bends to life's shifts rather than breaking.

Advocating for your liver health doesn't stop at personal choices. Sharing your experience and knowledge with loved ones extends the benefits further. Encourage friends or family to try a Mediterranean-style meal, discuss recipes, or organize group grocery trips. Even small acts of advocacy contribute to a more supportive environment for everyone navigating similar challenges.

Integrating structured planning, mindful tracking, and flexible food choices into your lifestyle anchors lifelong habits that safeguard liver health. Sustaining momentum is not about never straying from the plan, but about returning to a balanced routine and using every step forward or sideways as fuel for lasting change. With each cycle, adjustment, and reflection, you build a robust foundation for both your liver's vitality and your overall well-being.

FAQs

How can I adjust this meal plan for gluten intolerance or vegetarian preferences?

The 21-day liver-friendly meal plan is designed for flexibility and can be tailored for various dietary needs. For gluten intolerance, focus on naturally gluten-free Mediterranean staples like legumes, fresh vegetables, fruits, fish, poultry, and dairy. Swap out wheat-based grains (such as couscous or bulgur) for certified gluten-free options like quinoa, brown rice, or oats, and check labels to avoid hidden gluten.

For vegetarians, rely on plant-based proteins such as lentils, chickpeas, tofu, nuts, and seeds—substitute animal proteins in recipes with these alternatives. Including eggs and dairy expands your options. To ensure complete proteins, combine different legumes and grains (e.g., lentil pilafs or rice-and-bean salads). The plan's low-sugar focus remains attainable if you choose whole, minimally processed ingredients.

What are warning signs that my liver health isn't improving?

Liver issues can be subtle but watch for persistent fatigue, unexplained weakness, abdominal discomfort (especially in the upper right side), swelling in the legs or abdomen, or jaundice. Women with fatty liver should also note new digestive problems, easy bruising, or changes in mental clarity. Monitor shifts in energy, sleep, or menstrual cycles, as these can signal the need to reassess your plan or consult your doctor. Regularly track symptoms and use self-monitoring tools to catch concerns early.

Can I repeat the 21-day meal plan or should I add new recipes?

Repeating the 21-day cycle is safe and supports liver health if you maintain variety and stick to Mediterranean, low-sugar principles. Rotate core ingredients—leafy greens, legumes, olive oil, fish, poultry, nuts, and fresh fruits—to keep meals interesting. If you get bored, add new recipes within the same dietary framework. Focus on minimizing added sugars and processed foods, and use the guide's recipe-building tips to swap or introduce new dishes.

How do I increase meal variety without raising sugar intake?

Expand your menu by choosing low-glycemic vegetables (e.g., leafy greens, broccoli, bell peppers, beans) and lower-sugar fruits (like berries, kiwi, grapefruit, or green apples). Opt for whole grains such as quinoa or brown rice and check for added sugars. Use herbs, spices, citrus, and vinegar for flavor, and enjoy traditional Mediterranean dips and salads, which are typically low in sugar. Always review ingredient lists in condiments and pre-made items.

What if I experience digestive discomfort in the first week?

Initial digestive changes (bloating, gas) are common when increasing fiber. Gradually ramp up fiber-rich foods, stay hydrated, chew thoroughly, and lightly cook vegetables to aid digestion. If certain foods cause discomfort, reduce their portion or try alternatives. Consult your doctor if symptoms persist or worsen, especially for women with liver concerns.

Are supplements necessary for liver support?

The meal plan emphasizes food-first strategies. While some consider supplements like vitamin E or omega-3s, evidence is mixed. Always consult your physician before starting supplements, as some can interact with medications. A varied Mediterranean diet usually provides all needed nutrients.

How can I maintain social connections and dine out?

You can stay social by planning ahead: review menus for liver-friendly options, request dressings on the side, and bring dishes to gatherings. Opt for sparkling water with citrus instead of sugary drinks. If options are limited, do your best and return to your plan at the next meal. The Mediterranean diet encourages mindful eating and shared meals use these opportunities to enjoy food and company without stressing about perfection.

References and Helpful Links

Riazi, K., Azhari, H., Charette, J. et al.. (2022). The prevalence and incidence of NAFLD worldwide: a systematic review and meta-analysis. The Lancet Gastroenterology & Hepatology. https://doi.org/10.1016/s2468-1253(22)00165-0

Gawrieh, S., Chalasani, N.. (2018). Emerging Treatments for Nonalcoholic Fatty Liver Disease and Nonalcoholic Steatohepatitis. https://doi.org/10.1016/j.cld.2017.08.013

Ryan, M., Itsiopoulos, C., Thodis, T. et al.. (2013). The Mediterranean diet improves hepatic steatosis and insulin sensitivity in individuals with non-alcoholic fatty liver disease. Retrieved from https://doi.org/10.1016/j.jhep.2013.02.012

Vilar-Gomez, E., Martinez-Perez, Y., Calzadilla-Bertot, L. et al.. (2015). Weight Loss Through Lifestyle Modification Significantly Reduces Features of Nonalcoholic Steatohepatitis. https://doi.org/10.1053/j.gastro.2015.04.005

Morán-Costoya, A., Proenza, A., Gianotti, M. et al.. (2021). Sex Differences in Nonalcoholic Fatty Liver Disease: Estrogen Influence on the Liver–Adipose Tissue Crosstalk. Antioxidants & Redox Signaling. https://doi.org/10.1089/ars.2021.0044

Yki-Järvinen, H.. (2014). Non-alcoholic fatty liver disease as a cause and a consequence of metabolic syndrome. Retrieved from https://doi.org/10.1016/s2213-8587(14)70032-4

Farha, W., Abd El-Aty, A. M., Rahman, M. M., Jeong, J. H., Shin, H. C., Wang, J., ... & Shim, J. H.. (2018). Analytical approach, dissipation pattern and risk assessment of pesticide residue in green leafy vegetables: A comprehensive review.. Retrieved February 19, 2026, from https://analyticalsciencejournals.onlinelibrary.wiley.com/doi/abs/10.1002/bmc.4134

www.ingramcontent.com/pod-product-compliance
Lightning Source LLC
LaVergne TN
LVHW022230200926
848481LV00006B/2196
* 9 7 9 8 2 9 5 7 4 0 9 8 5 *